Reaching out to People in Comatose States

AF210264

RESEARCH SOCIETY FOR
PROCESS ORIENTED PSYCHOLOGY U.K.
c/o Interchange Studios, Hampstead Town Hall Centre,
213 Haverstock Hill, London NW3 4QP
Ltd. Co.: 4794982. Reg. Charity: 1107684

Reaching out
TO PEOPLE IN COMATOSE STATES
CONTACT AND COMMUNICATION

Peter Ammann

Diploma Thesis

Submitted to the Examination Board of the Faculty
in Partial Fulfillment of the Requirements for the Diploma in
Process-oriented Psychology
September 2010

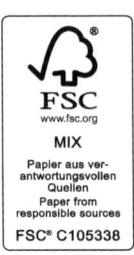

Cover design by Peter Ammann
Manufacturing and publishing house:
Books on Demand GmbH, Norderstedt

German Library Cataloguing in Publication Data
A catalogue record for this book is available from the German
Library:
http://dnb.d-nb.de.

ISBN 978-3-8448-1407-1

This book is alos available on the World Wide Web as an
eBook.

Printed in Germany

TABLE OF CONTENTS

LIST OF FIGURES

LIST OF TABLES

ACKNOWLEDGEMENTS

This diploma thesis owes its existence to the founder of Process Work Dr. Arnold Mindell and his colleagues. By the further development of Process Work and its application to people in comatose states Dr. Arnold Mindell with his wife Dr. Amy Mindell paved the way for applying this work on an intensive care unit and also in so many settings. I deeply appreciate Arny's and Amy's pioneering work, inspiring and heartful teaching and support over all these years.

For the beginning of this life-changing learning process and personal path 17 years ago I am indebted to my teachers Jean-Claude and Arlene Audergon. One of the most precious things I learned from them is a deep trust in nature which enabled me to trust in the potential for awareness even in the deepest altered states of consciousness.

I am also very grateful to Dr. Max Schüpbach for introducing me to the area of coma and dying and for showing me the potential for experiencing these states as moments of deep meaningful and completing realizations. Max's profound experience in world work and role theory helped me to see coma not simply as the experience of an individual but as a process in a field at the same time.

The openness and support of Prof. Dr. Irene Daum and her team at the Institute of Cognitive Neuroscience, Neuropsychology of the Ruhr-University Bochum enabled me to do this research in partial fulfillment of the requirements for my diploma in psychology. I am grateful to Dr. Boris Suchan my supervisor at university for his support and my second supervisor Dr. Denise Soria Bauser for her feedback and evaluation.

I am thankful to Prof. Dr. Helmut Hildebrandt and Prof. Dr. Andreas Zieger, both from the Carl von Ossietzky University Oldenburg, for their research activity on the subject of coma and Prof. Dr. Hildebrandt for placing the technical equipment at my disposal and for giving helpful advice.

Without the open mind and encouragement of Prof. Dr. Rolf Biniek at the hospital Rheinische Landesklinik Bonn, department of neurology and his team of physicians, nurses, physiotherapists, logotherapists, social workers, administrative assistants and cleaners I would not have had the opportunity to realize this research. I deeply acknowledge their support in inviting me into their everyday work and enabling me to gain insight into and understanding of other professions' endeavors in working with comatose patients.

I owe deep gratitude to all the patients I worked with for being able to make contact and to communicate in their unique way. I found myself challenged and sometimes blessed in following and guiding them through deep experiences at the edge of life and death. I learned such a lot from them, including about myself. I also deeply appreciate their relatives allowing me and trusting me to work with their loved ones.

Without the unwavering support, teaching, challenge and love of the community of the Research Society for Process-oriented Psychology U.K and visiting teachers, I would not have had the staying power and not have been able to carry out this project and the associated research. Especially I say thank you to my teachers, therapists, supervisors and study committee members: Jean-Claude Audergon, Arlene Audergon, Max Schüpbach, Jan Dworkin, Gary Reiss, Mark O'Connell and Anup Karia.

I am very thankful to Jan Webster from Coma Care, Cape Town for sharing, developing and learning together over a long period of time. I am most grateful to my friend and colleague on the "Traumland Intensivstation" project Thomas Kammerer, Catholic priest and member of the clinical pastoral care team of Ludwig-

Maximilian-University for his invaluable support.

I owe my fellow student Claire Seabrook a debt of gratitude for her endless stamina in editing this paper, for her precise thinking and utmost care. She has been a constant and reliable support; her presence and interest in my work and progress have helped me to bring this project to completion.

I feel deeply connected to my first wife Gundula and my mother Frieda, blessed by the relationships and experiences we had and strongly touched and moved by their going through coma, various altered states of consciousness and the dying process.

I owe special thanks to Kirsten Wassermann for her interest and support in this project and research. Without the intense and trans-forming long-term relationship we had I would not have developed the sensitivity and compassion to connect to these patients.

Finally my heart is with my children Kyra and Raphael who have been missing me from time to time when I was absorbed in my work.

This research is the result of a huge co-creation of people I have named and countless others who have contributed to it.

Peter Ammann
Wuppertal, Germany
September, 2010

FOREWORD

This paper is a revised and expanded version of the diploma thesis "Effects of Process-oriented Interventions in Comatose Patients" submitted for a postgraduate diploma in psychology at university. The concern of this continued effort is to add to this first explorative empirical research which comprised the application of Process-oriented Coma Work interventions to comatose patients on an intensive care unit, a survey of most relevant research in awareness of people in coma, vegetative state and minimally conscious state, a review of misdiagnosis and late recoveries of people in these altered states of consciousness, a philosophical and ethical discussion, an example of a comatose patient waking up through the use of Process-oriented Coma Work interventions and finally some personal experiences, reflections and insights.

1. INTRODUCTION

Coma confronts us with unsolved medical, ethically trouble-some and personally challenging situations. Medical advances have allowed more severely injured patients to survive and consequently the number of patients in the comatose, vegetative and minimally conscious state has proportionately increased. This frequently marginalized group of patients and their caregivers seldom gets a voice or support in society. Incidents of patients being removed from life support sometimes come to light as in the cases of Karen Ann Quinlan in 1985, Terri Schiavo in 2005 or Eluana Englaro in 2009. Some of the most important questions in these situations are: is there still consciousness in comatose people and can we contact them and communicate with them?

Should we talk and relate to comatose patients or should we maintain the attitude of talking "about" comatose patients as expressed by Posner et al. (2007, p. 7) in one of the standard works in neurology?

In contrast to this prevailing opinion Arnold Mindell (1989) assumes that coma is an extremely deep altered state and not an experience of unconsciousness, that comatose people are going through one more meaningful step in their process of individuation and that as Amy Mindell (1999, p. 28) says "if the heart is still beating, we should make the attempt to communicate and not rule out the possibility of reaching these little-known corners of life".

This first explorative study will investigate and test the effects of Process-oriented Coma Work interventions originated by Mindell and the assumptions on which they are based. Practical and ethical consequences will be discussed.

1.1   Coma and states related to or confused with coma

The nomenclature of disorders of consciousness has been developing and changing over the past 30 years (Giacino et al., 1995; Zasler, 2004). Terms have been used with different meanings not only among lay people but also in the professional field according to different areas of neuroscience and languages. New terms were defined but still are not used in all countries and also with different meanings. This chapter gives a short introduction and overview of the terms of coma and states related to or confused with coma which have a broad consensus in Western neuroscience at the time of writing.

1.1.1   Coma

Coma, from the Greek "κῶμα" meaning deep sleep or trance, is the deepest predominantly quantitative disorder of consciousness (Scharfetter, 1996). The medical definition of *coma* at present describes a comatose patient as lying down with eyes closed, not showing any sleep-wake cycles, and remaining in a state of unresponsiveness where he cannot be aroused to respond adequately to stimuli even with vigorous stimulation. The only responses to painful stimuli may be grimaces or stereotyped withdrawal responses of limbs. No localizing responses or discrete defensive movements appear.

In deeper stages of *coma* the responsiveness of the patient to even painful stimuli may diminish or disappear (Posner et al., 2007). According to the World Federation of Neurosurgeons (WFNS) *coma* is often classified into four different stages. Stage I implies unconsciousness without any further neurological symptoms. Through stages II to IV neurological symptoms increase, become deeper and more severe and central brain structures get involved such as the brainstem in the fourth stage (Leuwer et al., 2004; Hinder et al., 2001).

Coma may result from structural or metabolic changes. Structural damage can result from traumatic or non-traumatic sources.

Metabolic *coma* may result from a lack of substance, changes in neuronal electrical activity, disturbances in the balance of electrolytes, or complex multiple metabolic changes. Inflammations or infections can also cause general dysfunctions of both hemispheres (Hinder et al., 2001). The most important causes of *coma* are: hypoxic, cerebrovascular, metabolic and infections (Levy et al., 1981; Hamel et al., 1995; Thacker et al., 1997).

This kind of unconscious state rarely lasts for more than two to four weeks. Patients who do not recover from *coma* will either die or pass into a vegetative or minimally conscious state (Posner et al., 2007).

There is another condition in patients which appears like *coma* but is induced by pharmacological treatment (analgo-sedation) to support patients tolerating intubation or to treat pain caused by their medical condition or the treatment which is needed. The idea of using sedation in order to shield patients from anxiety and other emotional stress is currently under debate. That intentionally induced *"coma"* may sometimes be maintained for several weeks.

Coma does not only occur due to acute diseases or accidents but also often during the final days of life as part of the dying process. From a medical perspective people will lapse into coma in the end stages of liver, kidneys, lung failure, intracranial pressure or hypovolaemia (decrease in volume of blood plasma) (Bausewein et al., 2007; Ludwig, 2000).

1.1.2 Vegetative state

The Multi-Society Task Force on Persistent Vegetative State (MSTF) (part I, 1994) developed the diagnostic criteria for the *vegetative state* (VS). Like Posner et al. (2007) they see the *vegetative state* as a condition of complete unawareness of the self and the environment. Further characteristics are the return of so-called vegetative (autonomic) functions, including sleep-wake cycles, and normalization of respiratory and digestive system functions, potential for subcortical responses to external stimulation, including generalized physiologic responses to pain such as posturing, tachycardia, and diaphoresis, and subcortical motor responses, such as a grasp reflex. People in *vegetative state* show periods of eye opening and roving eye movements without concomitant visual tracking ability.

The symptoms of *vegetative state* were first described by W. Rosenblatt (1899, in Zasler, 2004) and concerned a man dying eight months after a concussion. Kretschmer (1940) gave a more detailed description of this state, classified it as a transitory condition and suggested the term "apallic syndrome" like Gerstenbrand (1967) in his monograph. But the term was not adopted in Anglo-American usage.

The term *"persistent vegetative state"* (PVS) was introduced for the first time by Jennet and Plum in 1972. They distinguished between the *persistent* and the *permanent vegetative state*. Although the *persistent vegetative state* was not associated with a specific duration of time, according to the American Neurological Association it is now applied only to patients in the state for one month (Celesia, 1993).

Although there are no clear criteria to say when the *persistent vegetative* becomes permanent, based on the data, the Multi-Society Task Force on PVS (part I and II, 1994) suggested that *vegetative state* after 12 months following traumatic brain injury (TBI), or 3 months following an anoxic injury, should be considered essentially permanent. The Royal College of Medicine in London (2003) however suggests a time frame of six months (see also Jennet, 2002). However, it is important to recognize that a small number of patients may recover from *vegetative state* beyond these time points (Rosenberg et al., 1977; Childs & Mercer, 1996; late remission in children: Heindl & Laub, 1996; Matsuda et al., 2003; Owen et al., 2007; Di et al., 2007).

The criteria for *permanent vegetative state* should be utilized for prognostic purposes relative to determining that emergence from *vegetative state* is statistically highly unlikely (Giacino et al., 1997, p. 81-82). There is an ongoing discussion about these terms and their practical and ethical consequences. The MSTF on PVS (1994) do not believe that the descriptor "persistent" and "permanent" clarify either the diagnosis or prognosis of the patient in the *vegetative state*.

During the International working party on the management of the *vegetative state* (Andrews, 1996) 16 experts agreed with each other on the inappropriateness of the term "persistent". W. Young even points out that the "introduction of the term *permanent vegetative state* serves only to create a self-fulfilling prophecy environment that surely does not encourage clinicians and scientists to pursue treatments that may ameliorate if not cure the condition" (1994, in Giacino et al., 1995, p. 43).

Other terms in the literature designating the *vegetative state* include coma vigil, coma depassé, post-coma unresponsiveness, and the apallic state.

1.1.3 Minimally conscious state

The term *minimally conscious state* (MCS) was developed in 1997 by the Aspen Neurobehavioral Conference Workgroup on VS and MCS, a consortium of neurologists, neurosurgeons, neuropsychologists, and rehabilitation specialists (Giacino et al., 1997).

They replaced the existing term minimally responsive state (MR) which was formulated by the Brain Injury Interdisciplinary Special Interest Group of the American Congress of Rehabilitation Medicine (1995) to emphasize that people's responses in *minimally conscious state* are consciously mediated and not reflexive or automatic.

Minimally conscious state identifies a condition of severely impaired consciousness in which minimal but definite behavioral evidence of self or environmental awareness is demonstrated. In order to define *minimally conscious state*, Giacino et al. (2002) carried out an evidence-based literature review of disorders of consciousness. They developed diagnostic criteria for entry into *minimally conscious state*, and identified markers for emergence to higher levels of cognitive functions.

Minimally conscious state often exists as a transitional state arising during recovery from coma, vegetative state or worsening of progressive neurologic disease. In some patients, however, it may be an essentially permanent condition but there are no data to allow guidelines for the expected duration of *minimally conscious state* (Posner et al., 2007, p. 363). On the contrary there are remissions after years. Voss' research (2006) suggests axonal regrowth underlying the process of a man emerging from *minimally conscious state* after 19 years.

Table 1. Comparison of clinical features associated with coma, vegetative state, minimally conscious state and locked-in syndrome (Giacino et al., 2002)

Condition	Consciousness	Sleep/Wake	Motor function
Coma	None	Absent	Reflex and postural responses only
Vegetative state	None	Present	Postures or withdraws to noxious stimuli
			Occasional nonpurposeful movement
Minimally conscious state	Partial	Present	Localizes noxious stimuli
			Reaches for objects
			Holds or touches objects in a manner that accommodates size and shape
			Automatic movements (e.g., scratching)
Locked-in syndrome	Full	Present	Quadri-phlegic

Auditory function	Visual function	Communication	Emotion
None	None	None	None
Startle	Startle	None	None
Brief orienting to sound	Brief visual fixation		Reflexive crying or smiling
Localizes sound location	Sustained visual fixation	Contingent vocalization	Contingent smiling or crying
Inconsistent command following	Sustained visual pursuit	Inconsistent but intelligible verbalization or gesture	
Preserved	Preserved	Aphonic/ Anarthric	Preserved
		Vertical eye movement and blinking usually intact	

1.1.4 Locked-in syndrome

Even though *locked-in syndrome* (LIS) is not a disorder of consciousness, due to the lesion of the ventral part of the brain stem (base and tegmentum of the midpons) that interrupts descending cortical control of motor functions, it is common for patients to experience an initial coma or to respond inconsistently in the beginning, in a similar way to minimally conscious state. This de-efference results in paralysis of all four limbs and the lower cranial nerves. Patients in *locked-in syndrome* usually retain control of vertical eye movement and eyelid opening.

The Guillain-Barré syndrome (GBS) may have a similar appearance but has a history of sub acute paralysis. Both conditions disclose a reactive posterior alpha rhythm in the encephalographic (EEG) examination.

The symptoms of *locked-in syndrome* have been observed since the 19th century, but the distinctive name was applied in the first edition of "The Diagnosis of Stupor and Coma" by F. Plum and J. B. Posner (1966). There are reports of 5-, 10-, and 20 years survival. Self-scored perception of mental health and personal general health were not significantly lower than values from age-matched control subjects (Posner et al., 2007, p. 363).

1.1.5 Psychogenic unresponsiveness

The definition and explanatory model of *psychogenic unresponsiveness* used in neurology originate from a psychoanalytical point of view. *Psychogenic unresponsiveness* is quite uncommon and psychogenic coma is even more rare.

Nevertheless to diagnose *psychogenic unresponsiveness* among all other psychogenic illnesses that mimic structural disease is very challenging. Sometimes a structural disease is initially diagnosed as psychogenic and sometimes the other way round. The latter occurs especially when psychogenic coma complicates a structural illness as a reaction or psychological defense against it. If a patient having a severe organic illness becomes unresponsive the examiner may fail to keep in mind that the unresponsiveness is psychogenic and represents for example a conversion reaction to a difficult psychological situation. Several tests can help to differentiate between structural and psychogenic unresponsiveness (Posner et al., 2007; Cartlidge, 2001).

Several psychiatric disorders may result in *psychogenic unresponsiveness*. The cause of most psychogenic unresponsiveness is a conversion reaction, a psychogenic or non-physiologic loss of neurologic function involving the special senses or the voluntary nervous system. It may occur as a psychological defense or a reaction to organic disease. Secondly there is catatonic stupor which is a symptom complex characterized by either stupor or excitement accompanied by behavioral disturbances that include for example mutism, posturing, rigidity, grimacing, waxy flexibility, and catalepsy. Thirdly there is dissociative or "fugue" state and fourthly sometimes factitious disorder or malingering.

Most unresponsive disorders come from a conversion reaction and others from the syndrome of catatonia (often thought to be a manifestation of schizophrenia). Even though most neurological routine tests like MRI, evoked potentials, and EEG are usually normal, measurement of cerebral metabolism is regionally abnormal (Posner et al., 2007).

Sleeping Beauty syndrome is another form of *psychogenic unresponsiveness* in children as a response to an extreme psychological impact for example after a severe accident with brain injury (Todorow, 1975, 1978). It appears as an apathetic-akinetic-mutistic state which transforms by continuous loving and related contact.

1.2 Assessing consciousness

The concept of consciousness has been a challenge for various scientific disciplines for centuries. On the one hand it is so familiar to us and on the other, its intimate nature eludes any attempt at a clear definition. Most definitions of consciousness in neuroscience follow approaches like those of neurologists Stanley Cobb (1952) or J. B. Posner et al. (2007), defining consciousness as the state of full awareness of the self and one's relationship to the environment. Such a definition is unable to resist the reproach of being tautological (Avanzini, 1999).

A more in-depth discussion about the concept and its consequences follows in a subsequent chapter.

In the field of neuroscience, consciousness is often pragmatically reduced to either two components: content and arousal (Posner et al., 2007) or three: vigilance (alertness), mental contents, and selective attention (Niedermeyer, 1999). Furthermore two sources of information are distinguished: overt and covert behavior. Overt behavior can be perceived from the outside and exists in verbal expressions or any other noticeable signal in various sensory modes, whereas covert behavior can be observed indirectly only as physiological measurements and precedes overt behavior (Zieger & Hildebrandt, 1996).

1.2.1 Coma scales and scoring systems

Standardized systems to assess the level of consciousness use overt behavior and are divided into two categories: coma scales and coma scoring systems. Representative of the first category are: Rancho Los Amigos Scale (Hagen et al., 1979), Coma/Near-coma Scale (CNC) (Rappport et al., 1982) or Reaction Level Scale-85 (RLS-85) (Stalhammar & Starmark, 1986). The prototype, most known and widely used, in the second category of coma scoring systems is the Glasgow Coma Scale (GCS) (Teasdale & Jennett, 1974). Its name is misleading because it is not a scale by definition. A more elaborated one is the Comprehensive Level of Consciousness

Scale (CLOGS) (Stanczak et al., 1984). The Full Outline of UnResponsiveness (FOUR) (Wijdicks et al., 2005) is a new scoring system designed to potentially replace the GCS. These two categories of assessment of the level of consciousness arise from different assumptions and intentions.

The idea of a scale system is that functional changes and brain dysfunctions are correlated and therefore significant clinical signs fall into fixed patterns indicative of progressive brain dysfunction. It is a constellation of symptoms or pattern which is expressed in the "level" or "step" of the scale, whereas the assumption of a scoring system is that all symptoms or signs are independent. That is why the signs are gathered in categories and hierarchically arranged according to progressive functional impairment. Coma scoring systems are designed to assess the depth of coma, to predict prognosis and to monitor changes on examination (Bozza Marrubini, 1984; Spittler et al., 1993).

1.2.2 The Glasgow Coma Scale

Since the Glasgow Coma Scale (GCS) is applied in this research it will be described in more detail. The GCS is presently the most widely known and accepted assessment of level of consciousness. The GCS is typically used following traumatic brain injury, cerebrovascular accidents, cerebral infections, and metabolic disorders that have an effect on level of arousal. It takes less than five minutes to perform and is usually performed by trained health professionals, trauma team, or neurological or neurosurgical staff. The scale covers the present, serial measurements are useful in monitoring changes in level of consciousness. Because of its high validity claims it is applied in most research in the area of disorders of consciousness although it is strictly speaking not designed for assessing intubated and aphasic patients (Hinder et al., 2001).

Characteristics:

1. The scale categorizes three clinical examination findings: best **E**ye response, best **V**erbal response, and best **M**otor response.

- Each parameter is scored separately, the worst possible score in each case being 1, the best being 4 (for best eye-opening response), 5 (for best verbal response), or 6 (for best motor response).
- The three scores are combined to give a total score (range 3–15). Low scores indicate greater impairment of level of consciousness.
- The score is most helpfully reported as its component parts and as the total – e.g., E4, V3, M5, total 12/15 to retain differentiating information.
- Coma is defined by maximum score of 7 points or less. Patients with 8 points are also seen as comatose if they do not open their eyes after a painful stimulation (Hinder et al., 2001).

Even though the GCS is widely adopted it should not be overlooked that this scoring system has quite a few **shortcomings**:

- Many comatose patients are intubated and sometimes aphasic but the GCS is a priori not applicable for sedated or aphasic patients. (Hinder et al., 2001).
- Important aspects reflecting the severity of coma like abnormal brainstem reflexes, changing of breathing pattern, and the need for mechanical ventilation are not included.
- The GCS is not sensitive enough to monitor changes in neurological examination.
- The assessment of difference in light disorders of consciousness is reduced.

(Wijddicks et al., 2005; Spittler et al., 1993; Nijenhuis & de Vetten, 2006)

Table 2. Glasgow Coma Scale (Teasdale & Jennett, 1974)

Eye Response (E)	eyes open spontaneously	4
	eye opening to verbal command	3
	eye opening to pain	2
	no eye opening	1
Motor response (M)	obeys commands	6
	localizing pain	5
	withdrawal from pain	4
	flexion response to pain	3
	extension response to pain	2
	No motor response	1
Verbal Response (V)	oriented	5
	confused	4
	inappropriate words	3
	incomprehensible words	2
	no verbal response	1
Total Score (E+M+V)		3-15

1.3 Neurophysiologic correlates of consciousness and covert behavior in comatose states

Kolb & Whishaw (2003) describe four processes as prerequisites of consciousness: 1. arousal, 2. perception, 3. attention and 4. working memory. In neurology coma is traditionally understood as the decoupling of the reticular activating system (RAS), localized in the brain stem, from cortical and subcortical (thalamic) structures. The denervation of thalamic nuclei and of the cortex of the reticular activating system impulses leads to coma or coma vigile.

From the results of their various studies Hildebrandt et al. (1998 and 1999) understood coma as a decoupling of endogenuous brain stem rhythms of phasic activity states of different compartments of the nervous system. Their results make the process of emerging from coma appear a successive increase of the sympathetic activity and a reintegration of the sympathovagal balance. This pattern was demonstrated as integrated parameters in the power spectra of heart rate variability, variability of the electromyography of frontal muscles and variability of electrodermal activity.

Electrodermal activity expressed in skin conductance level (SCL) as tonic activation marker and in skin conductance responses (SCR) as phasic activation markers revealed significant changes. SCL values, SCR values and variability of SCR increased during the process of awakening from coma. In general, SCL and SCR increased with higher Glasgow Coma Score values. Therefore they suggest the use of these parameters as measurable covert behavior for a systematic analysis of different coma rehabilitation programs.

1.4   Electrodermal activity

Electrodermal activity (EDA) refers to all measurable changes in bioelectric activity of the skin which is physically describable such as changes in conductance, resistance or potential. First evidence of electrodermal activity was documented in 1888 by Féré (Boucsein, 1988). Interference from psychological factors was discovered around the same time.

1.4.1   Terminology

Recommendations of the Society for Psychophysiological Research helped to standardize various nomenclatures of electrodermal activity. According to them "S" stands for skin, "P" for potential, "R" for resistance, "C" for conductance, "Y" for admittance and "Z" for impedance.

Furthermore it is differentiated into tonic aspects "L" (level) and phasic aspects "R" (response). Correspondingly all tonic aspects of electrodermal activity (EDA) are referred to as EDL (electrodermal level) and all phasic aspects as EDR (electrodermal response).

As shown in Table 3 all methods of recording can be divided, first into endosomatic or exosomatic recordings and second in applied direct current (DC) or alternating current (AC). Under direct current, skin conductance (skin conductance level [SCL], skin conductance response [SCR]) or skin resistance (SRL/SRR) can be recorded (for more information sees Boucsein, 1988). In most studies and also in this one the skin conductance is applied.

Table 3. Nomenclature of electrodermal activity (Boucsein, 1988)

Methods of recording	endo-somatic	exo-somatic			
Applied current	none	direct current		alternating current	
Units	Skin potential	Skin conduc-tance	Skin resistance	Skin admit-tance	Skin impe-dance
Abbreviations:					
in general	SP	SC	SR	SY	SZ
tonic (level), EDL	SPL	SCL	SRL	SYL	SZL
phasic (response), EDR	SPR	SCR	SRR	SYR	SZR

(SP=skin potential, SC=skin conductance, SR=resistance, SY=skin admittance, SZ=skin impedance, SPL=skin potential level, SCL=skin conductance level, SRL=skin resistance level, SYL=skin admittance level, SZL=skin impedance level, SPR=skin potential response, SCR=skin conductance response, SRR=resistance response, SYR=skin admittance response, SZR=skin impedance response, EDL=electrodermal level, EDR=electrodermal response)

1.4.2 Skin and sweat glands

The skin fulfills two main functions: it separates and connects the body and the environment; protection and sensation are essential tasks. Furthermore adaptation processes such as release of water and the control of temperature play an important role (Gramann & Schandry, 2009).

Regarding the electrodermal activity the eccrine sweat glands whose main function consists of thermoregulation by sweating play the most important role. The eccrine sweat glands are composed of (1) an intraepidermal spiral duct, the "acrosyringium" (2) a straight dermal portion, and (3) a coiled acinar portion in the dermis or hypodermis, and are found at virtually all sites on the human body. The highest concentration of more than 2,000 per cm^2 can be found on palms and soles. The activity of sweat glands is controlled by the sympathetic aspect of the autonomic nervous system (ANS) and in contrast to other sympathetic activity the transmitter at postganglionic synapse for the sweat glands is not adrenalin or noradrenalin but acetylcholine. Due to the influence of sympathetic activity sweat glands react also very sensitively to emotional stimuli. Phasic aspects of electrodermal activity are seen as the most reliable and valid indicator of an orienting response (OR) (Vossel & Zimmer, 1998).

1.4.3   Skin conductance

According to modern models of electrodermal activity the sweat gland ducts act like resistors in parallel in a circuit. Depending on the sympathetic activity the sweat in ducts of sweat glands increases. With increased sweating the electrical resistance reduces and the conductance increases. Therefore every change in the amount of sweat in the ducts changes the values of the variable resistors. The addition of all single conductivity values results in the overall conductivity. The more simple measurement of conductivity lead the prevailing use of skin conductance compared with skin resistance (Boucsein, 1988).

Skin conductance is characterized by tonic (SCL) and phasic changes (SCR). Skin conductance is usually measured today in "Siemens" (S) units. As the conductivity of the skin is very small, values are usually given in micro Siemens ($\mu S/cm^2$). Slow modulation of skin conductance level (SCL) varies in a range from 2 to 100 $\mu S/cm^2$, frequently between 5 and 20 $\mu S/cm^2$. Changes of values often occur within a time frame of 10 to 30 seconds. Levels and dynamics of skin conductance vary from one individual to another. Within (and largely independent of) these different SCL levels, many sharp peaks in skin conductance occur.

These short modulations in the signal are phasic phenomena and each peak represents an individual skin conductance response (SCR) to a stimulus (orienting response). An SCR is a discrete and short fluctuation in skin conductance that lasts several seconds and usually follows a characteristic pattern of an initial, relatively steep rise, a short peak, and then a relatively slower return to baseline.

SCRs reflect the higher-frequency variability of the signal that is modulated on top of the slower changes in SCL. Skin conductance responses vary between 0.02 and 0.1 $\mu S/cm^2$ (Vossel & Zimmer, 1998).

Figure 2 shows a measurement of skin conductance where tonic and phasic aspects of skin conductance can be seen. From the beginning to the 55th second the SCL varies between 2.0 and 2.5 $\mu S/cm^2$. Within this time small fluctuations in skin conductance level (SCL), skin conductance responses (SCR) such as marked in "R" can be seen.

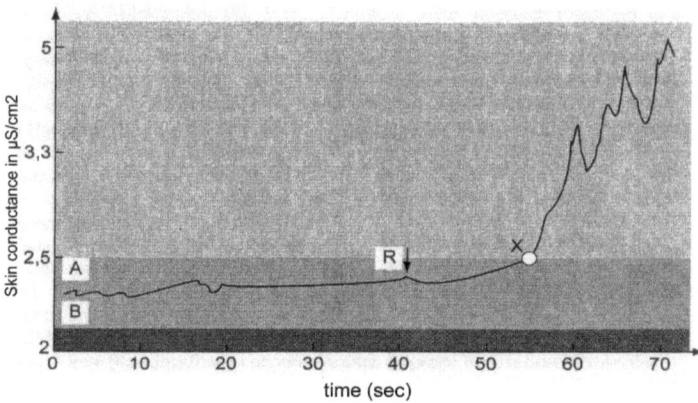

Figure 1. Skin conductance curve (A, B = upper and lower level of range, R=Response)

Changes in level (SCL) as well as the number of spontaneous reactions (SCR) provide information about activation. Substantial correlations between the frequency and intensity of electrodermal changes and the frequency of sympathetic action potentials are documented (Wallin, 1981). While the central origins of the autonomic nervous system are within the hypothalamus and the brainstem,

17

other parts of the brain such as the amygdala, the hippocampus, the basal ganglia, and the prefrontal cortex, have been found to be involved in the control of eccrine sweating.

These "higher" areas are part of the limbic and paralimbic networks, which are crucially involved in affective processes. Thus it is not surprising that skin conductance is often used as an indicator of emotional arousal and other affective processes. Interestingly, it has been shown that these higher brain areas are not involved for reflex SCRs to non-emotional stimuli such as deep breaths and orienting stimuli such as a loud noise, but they are necessary for SCRs in response to stimuli that have acquired emotional value through experience, e.g. in classical conditioning (Naqvi & Bechara, 2006; Tranel & Damasio, 1994).

1.5   Comatose and vegetative state patients' ability to hear

People's ability to hear even in comatose states has been investigated by varying methods such as auditory brain-stem response (ABR), event-related potentials (ERP) and neuroimaging techniques.

Hearing as a processing of auditory information can be roughly distinguished into two stages, sometimes also referred to sensation and perception. Changes of air pressure are detected by receptors in the inner ear; action potentials are conveyed via neural pathway to the brain and reach the primary cortices. In the next stage primary cortices relay signals to adjacent areas which are referred to as secondary cortices and thought to be more engaged in interpreting perceptions. Further areas in between various secondary areas are called tertiary cortices or associative cortices. These tertiary areas serve to connect and coordinate the function of the secondary areas, and perform complex activities such as language, planning, memory, and attention (Kolb & Wishaw, 2003).

Yagi & Baba (1983) investigated auditory brain-stem responses (ABRs) and caloric vestibular reactions (CVRs) in 100 deep comatose patients to evaluate the brain-stem function of these patients and to predict their prognosis. Auditory brain-stem responses performed within 24-48 hours after the onset of deep coma and later on, were evoked by 110 dB SPL (sound pressure level) click stimuli alternating in polarity with interstimulus intervals of 75 ms presented through headphones monaurally.

The auditory brain-stem responses were recorded between the vertex or the center of the forehead near the hairline, and the ipsilateral mastoid or earlobe. The contralateral mastoid or earlobe was grounded.

Among other results 54 of 100 comatose patients showed normal and 46 abnormal auditory brain-stem responses. Among the latter, 21 exhibited no auditory brain-stem responses.

Event-related brain potentials (ERPs) are another noninvasive method of studying the neurophysiology and elements of consciousness. ERPs are brief changes, waves time-locked to particular events like sensory stimulus or a patient's motor response in an electroencephalogram (EEG).

The latency of event-related brain potentials corresponds to the successive activation of many regions of the brain by a stimulus. Early cortical components, up to about 100 milliseconds designate processes in primary cortex regions where those appearing from 100 to 300 milliseconds after the stimulus designate more secondary and tertiary regions of the cortex and are likely to be related to the meaning of a stimulus. Waves appearing 300 milliseconds after stimulus presentation, referred to as P300 or P_{3}, are thought to represent the process of decoding the meaning of the sounds (Kolb & Whishaw, 2003).

Studies from Fischer et al. (1999), Gott et al. (1991), Guerit et al. (1999), Kane et al. (2000) and Mutschler et al. (1996) already demonstrated the ability of the coma patient's cortex to differentiate between frequent and rare events in simple sine tones (an estimate of 30-50%). Kotchoubey et al. (2002) investigated event-related brain potentials in 34 patients (17 in *vegetative state* and 17 in minimally conscious state) presenting sine tones, complex tones and vowels in an oddball paradigm in which rare (e.g., 20%) stimuli ("targets") are randomly inserted in a sequence of frequent (e.g., 80%) stimuli and the subjects' task is usually to count the rare events

Summarizing the results, one- to two thirds of patients with suspected vegetative state were capable of cortical differentiation of physical stimulus features and at least 20% of these patients also differentiated semantic stimuli. That means their brains obviously comprehended language.

In order to evaluate the differences in brain activation in response to presentation of the patient's own name spoken by a familiar voice in patients with vegetative state and minimally conscious state, Di et al. (2007) used fMRI in severely brain-damaged patients. Five of seven patients in vegetative state did show significant activation within auditory cortices. Two of these five patients showed even more widespread activation not only in Heschl's gyrus (HG) but extending to the planum temporale, the planum polare, and the posterior and lateral extensions of HG as associative auditory cortices.

This research also confirms PET studies by Laureys et al. (2000a) and Boly et al. (2004) on simple auditory stimuli eliciting group-level activation in the primary auditory cortex of patients in vegetative state.

These results derived from different methods clearly demonstrate that higher cortical functions are preserved in many patients who cannot express their abilities in their overt behavior.

1.6 Reports from patients after a period of unconsciousness

"We know each other, doctor, but you never say hello to me. Why do you act as if I'm not here?" is one of the thoughts a college student recalled who recovered from severe anoxic encephalopathy after coming out of 53 days of coma (Steuck, 1978). This is one of many recollections and reported experiences of people who emerged from a coma, vegetative state or minimally conscious state. In addition to these anecdotal accounts and in contrast to prevailing medical or neuropsychological, third-person research approaches, several systematic studies were conducted to explore occurrences during coma or unconsciousness from the perspective of the patient in retrospect.

Schnaper (1975) informally interviewed 68 patients, selected on the basis of recovery of consciousness and availability over a 12-month period, to explore psychological implications of severe trauma including defense mechanism. 43 patients of this group (63%) claimed amnesia at the time of the interview. A second group of eight patients (12%) pleaded amnesia but subsequently were able to recall the experience. A third group of 17 patients (25%) recalled experiences from the period of unconsciousness. The prevailing themes of the second and third group together were fantasies and experiences of being held prisoner, wrongdoing to justify imprisonment, and death.

In a replication of Schnaper's study, Tosch (1988) explored recollections of post-traumatic coma viewed retrospectively by the patient after regaining consciousness and prior to discharge from the hospital. Coma was defined as GCS score of less than or equal to 8 for at least six hours. The sample consisted of fifteen adult patients of two hospitals who had regained consciousness after incurring a head injury and related post-traumatic coma. Data were collected during face-to-face meetings using a semi-structured interview. Eleven patients (73%) initially claimed amnesia; four of these subsequently were able to recall experiences and seven subjects remained amnestic. The other group of eight subjects (53%) were able to relate experiences with three prevailing themes: imprisonment (being held against their will), sensory experiences (intensified visual, olfactory or auditory perception), and death-like experiences. Patients with post-traumatic coma of more than ten days' duration had a greater tendency for amnesia compared to those subjects who remained in post-traumatic coma for less than ten days. Recollections of experiences during the period of unconsciousness were not correlated with the GCS score or type of head injury sustained but with the length of coma.

Another research question concerned patients' recollections of actions helpful or not helpful to them. Four out of 15 patients (27%) found physical touch, hearing details of the accident and reassuring voices helpful. Three patients also recalled painful pinches (20%) (including one patient remembering nipple pinches [which is luckily not practiced anymore]) and angry voices not being helpful and unpleasant.

As a follow up of Podurgiel's (1990) pilot study involving eleven unconscious patients in hospital, Lawrence (1995) carried out a descriptive study exploring the states patients experienced during a period of documented unconsciousness. 100 patients were interviewed face-to-face in an unstructured interview after regaining consciousness. The data were classified as five types of altered consciousness experiences and resulted in the following distribution: 1. Unconsciousness (27%), 2. Inner consciousness (9%), 3. Perceived unconsciousness (auditory, tactile, emotional, movement; 27%), 4. Distorted consciousness (perceptual distortion, memory distortion, personality distortion; 14%), and 5. Paranormal experiences (such as near-death experiences, out-of-body experiences, near-death visits and encounter with the Grim Reaper; 23%).

Rundshagen et al. (2002) conducted a prospective clinical study to investigate the incidence of recall and dreams during analgo-sedation in 289 critically ill patients who either arrived intubated and sedated at the intensive care unit (ICU) or required intubation, mechanical ventilation, and sedation during their ICU stay. Patients were interviewed with a structured interview within 48-72 hours after discharge from the ICU if they recalled any event or dreams before they regained consciousness. Results showed 187 (65%) who did not remember anything during the period of unconsciousness, whereas another group of 49 (17%) patients recalled experiences from this period. A smaller group of patients (21%) remembered dreams from the period between loss of consciousness and regaining it.

All the above studies demonstrate strong evidence for consciousness in so-called unconscious states. Findings of these and further studies such as reports of unpleasant experiences of ICU patients (Turner et al., 1990), documentation of high incidence of recall for the respirator treatment (Bergbohm-Engberg et al., 1989), exploratory study of patient's perception, memories and experiences of an ICU (Russell, 1999), or findings of very high incidences for night-mares in survivors of the acute respiratory distress syndrome (Schelling et al., 1998) are varying in the design, using unstructured interviews or standard questionnaire, sometimes lacking information about the regimes of sedation and not being sure when exactly at what time or stage memories occurred, but all of them are demonstrating a strong tendency of a high evidence for awareness in so-called unconscious states.

Several studies mention patients' hesitation about sharing or even remembering these experiences out of anxiety about being stigmatized as crazy which mirrors a cultural marginalization of altered states of consciousness. Recent studies have explored themes already discussed to some extent by La Puma (1988) for example that not talking to comatose patients may promulgate the notion that these patients are dead or nearly dead, or that talking to comatose patients may benefit both doctor and patient. Furthermore feedback from patients reveals that personal contact and warmth, being called by name, being talked to and being cared about may increase the level of consciousness, may prevent psychological problems after discharge from the ICU and may increase the chance of survival of unconscious clients.

1.7 Misdiagnosis of vegetative state and minimally conscious state

The assessment of consciousness in people with disorders of consciousness is a challenging task for various reasons. Giacino & Zasler (1995) have pointed out the limitations of clinical assessment in the identification of "internal awareness" in patients who lack the motor functions to demonstrate their awareness. Schnakers et al. (2009) mentioned further difficulties such as the presence of tracheotomy, fluctuating arousal level or ambiguous and rapidly habituating responses. The consequences have a heavy impact on daily management, particularly in pain treatment, level of care or service provided, end-of-life decision-making (such as withdrawal of tube feeding and hydration) and prognosis (Andrews, 2004).

Four studies have surveyed diagnostic accuracy in respect of vegetative and minimally conscious states in recent years and showed up to 43% of misdiagnosis.

Tresch et al. (1991) assessed pre-admission diagnosis of long-term persistent vegetative state patients in a nursing home. They discovered 11 out of 62 persistent vegetative state patients (18%) being aware of themselves or their environment.

Childs et al. (1993) reviewed 193 severely brain-injured patients admitted for inpatient neurorehabilitation within a period of five years. 49 patients were at least one month post-injury and carried the diagnosis of persistent vegetative state or coma (in terms of vegetative state). 18 (37%) of these patients were diagnosed inaccurately.

Three years later Andrews et al. (1996) assessed 40 patients who had been admitted between 1992 and 1995 with a referral diagnosis of vegetative state. 17 patients (43%) were considered as having been misdiagnosed. Seven of these patients had been presumed to be in vegetative state for longer than a year, including three for over four years. In six weeks where they were examined and received occupational therapy, all of them were able to correctly answer simple biographical questions that required a yes/no response, for example using movements to press a simple touch-sensitive switch and also demonstrated other evidence of awareness.

In order to compare consensus-based diagnoses of vegetative state and minimally conscious state to those based on a standardized neurobehavioral rating scale, Schnakers et al. (2009) assessed 103 patients (collected between October 2005 and January 2007). Out of 44 patients with a clinical consensus diagnosis of vegetative state, 18 patients (41%) showed signs of awareness. In patients with pre-admission diagnosis of minimally conscious state (n=41), 10% (n=4) met criteria for emergence from minimally conscious state.

Despite the importance of diagnostic accuracy, the growing consistency of the nomenclature, and the development of specialized neurobehavioral rating scales to provide a reliable and valid means of detecting signs of consciousness, the rate of misdiagnosis of vegetative state has not substantially changed in the past 13 years!

Researchers involved in these studies, Zasler (2004) and also Laureys (2007) suggest various reasons for this situation. At the time of the first three studies, a lack of consistency in understanding the nomenclature, a lack of knowledge regarding the basic conditions and methods to evaluate and classify people in low-level-neurological states might have been relevant. Reliance on bedside observations by physicians rather than having a multidisciplinary team experienced in the management of people with complex disabilities, including family members, and taking into consideration various circumstances of the patient might have contributed to this high percentage of misdiagnosis. Diagnosis determined by clinical consensus instead of standardized neurobehavioral assessment could also have yielded this high rate of misdiagnosis. Extended observation for behavioral evidence of cognitive awareness by qualified personnel is seldom standard. In consequence subtle signs like purposeful eye movements, periods of higher arousal or body positions that enhance wakefulness are overlooked in the examination process.

Schnakers's (2009) recent findings and the fact that most of the reasons for misdiagnosis mentioned above have been known for a long time and that the nomenclature and methods of investigation have noticeably improved, may suggest that we still marginalize this group of patients.

1.8 Studies on evidence of consciousness in coma, vegetative state and minimally conscious state

Evidence of consciousness derived from assessing overt behavior has already been mentioned in patients' retrospective reports after a period of unconsciousness and by the disclosure of misdiagnosis in vegetative state patients. Unconscious patients' ability to hear, demonstrated by auditory brain-stem responses, P_3, waves in event-related brain potentials and activation of associative cortices are further evidence of consciousness and examples of covert behavior.

Investigation of the neural basis and evidence of consciousness in the late 1980s and 1990s was focused on studying the brain's electrical activity and event-related potentials such as heart rate variability, electrodermal activity and electromyography. Reuter et al. (1989) demonstrated cognitive potentials in patients in vegetative state in the form of P_3, waves. Szirtes et al. (1990) were able to show significant changes in the EEG power spectrum to semantic word potentials in vegetative state patients in reaction to the word "Mama". Zieger & Hildebrandt (1996) recorded significant changes in heart rate variability, electromyography and electrodermal activity during dialogic interventions with 23 comatose patients.

Further technical development using X-ray enabled scientists to look into the brain and to produce static two-dimensional images (conventional radiography, pneumoencephalography, angiography and computerized tomography). The next technical improvement allowed them to take three-dimensional images and to see brain structures more precisely and in function during activation. Positron-emission tomography (PET) and different kinds of magnetic resonance imaging (MRI), including functional magnetic resonance imaging (fMRI), became central to further investigation of consciousness in disorders of consciousness.

PET studies in vegetative state patients have consistently demonstrated diffuse, uniformly reduced cerebral metabolic activity (Schiff et al., 2002). However studies also revealed patients emerging from vegetative state without any considerable increase of cerebral metabolic activity and healthy people having a similar reduced activity to patients in vegetative state. Nevertheless in some cases people in vegetative state show a nearly normal activity. In contrast to the overall cerebral blood flow, regional changes of metabolism, especially in associative cortices, reveal big differences. In a state of awareness these cortices communicate with each other as well as with deeper brain structures, especially the thalamus (Laureys, 2004, 2008).

Laureys et al. (2000b) studied brain activations, measured by PET, in a vegetative state patient. Responses to simple auditory and somatosensory stimuli were restricted to the primary sensory cortices for both types of stimulus when compared with the baseline resting conditions. When the patient had recovered, fMRI showed the thalamocortical modulation was no longer different from controls.

In another study (Laureys et al., 2000a) PET was used to investigate regional cerebral blood flow in response to auditory stimulation in five vegetative state patients. Auditory click stimuli activated bilateral auditory cortices but not the contralateral auditory association cortices as they did in healthy controls. Moreover, the auditory association cortex was functionally disconnected from the posterior parietal association area, the anterior cingulated cortex and the hippocampus.

A further study of the Coma Science Group (Laureys et al., 2002) explored the experience of pain in vegetative state and healthy volunteers. Both groups demonstrated neuronal activity in the brain stem, thalamus and primary somatosensory cortices, but in vegetative state patients no other cortices reacted as they did in healthy volunteers.

These results suggest that the experience of pain of patients in vegetative state differs from that in healthy people. Another study, however, using a similar methodology in seven vegetative state patients contradicts this assumption. Kassubek et al. (2003) demonstrated activation not only in primary but also in secondary somatosensory, insular and anterior cingulated cortices in this PET study. Pain as a first-person experience remains controversial.

Schiff et al. (2002) identified evidence of partially functional cerebral regions in catastrophically injured brains. They studied five patients in vegetative state with different behavioral features and employed PET, MRI and magnetoencephalographic (MEG) to measure responses to sensory stimulation. In three of five patients, co-registered PET/MRI correlate islands of relatively preserved brain metabolism with isolated fragments of behavior. These behavioral fragments appear to consist of segregated corticothalamic networks that retain connectivity and partial functional integrity. This reflects evidence of the modular nature of individual functional networks that underlie conscious brain functions.

In order to test the hypothesis that minimally conscious state patients retain active cerebral networks that underlie cognitive function even though their reactions and communication abilities are fluctuating, Schiff et al. (2005) investigated two patients in minimally conscious state. They employed fMRI to evaluate cortical responses to passive language and tactile stimulation. In both cases these patients showed similar reactions in the primary sensory cortices and in high-order brain processing. The only difference to healthy volunteers appeared when the narratives were presented as a time-reversed signal, and therefore without linguistic content.

These findings may suggest defining vegetative state as a condition where human brains react to stimuli only automatically and only within the somatosensory primary cortices.

However Owen et al. (2006, 2007) detected evidence of awareness and intentionality in a patient who fulfilled all the criteria for a diagnosis of vegetative state according to international guidelines.

They used fMRI to measure her neural responses during a presentation of spoken sentences (e.g. "There was milk and sugar in his coffee.") which were compared with responses to acoustically matched noise sequences. Speech-specific activation was observed bilaterally in the middle and superior temporal gyri equivalent to that observed in healthy volunteers listening to the same stimuli. To test speech comprehension sentences that contained ambiguous words (italicized) (e.g., "The *creak* came from a *beam* in the *ceiling*.") were presented. fMRI showed an additional activation in the left inferior frontal region which is associated with semantic processing.

For further exploration of conscious awareness they conducted another fMRI study where the same patient was given spoken instructions to perform two mental imagery tasks at specific points during the scan. The first instruction "imagine playing tennis" revealed significant activity in the supplementary motor area; the second instruction "imagine visiting the rooms in your home" showed significant activity in the parahippocampal gyrus, posterior parietal cortex, and lateral premotor cortex. Activation patterns in both conditions were indistinguishable from those observed in healthy volunteers. In a third condition, the patient was asked to "just relax".

Despite her fulfilling all the clinical criteria for a diagnosis of being in vegetative state, they concluded that this patient retained the ability to understand spoken commands and to respond to them through her brain activity rather than through speech or movement.

Building on the study described above, Monti et al. (2010) used these two mental-imagery tasks and functional magnetic resonance imaging (fMRI) in 54 patients with disorders of consciousness (23 in a vegetative and 31 in minimal conscious state) and 16 healthy control subjects for two main aims. The first aim was to investigate to what extent patients could also reliably and repeatedly "willfully modulate" (author's quotation marks) their functional MRI responses, reflecting preserved awareness. The second aim was to develop and validate a method that would allow such patients to functionally communicate yes-or-no responses by "modulating" their own brain activity, without training and without the need for any motor response.

In the first part of this research all patients and healthy control subjects were given the motor imagery task ("Imagine standing still on a tennis court and swinging an arm to 'hit the ball' back and forth."), the spatial imagery task ("Imagine navigating the streets of a familiar city or imagine walking from room to room in your home and visualize all that you would 'see' if you were there.") or the instruction to relax. In the second phase of the experiment one patient who had reliable responses during the imagery tasks and sixteen controls were asked to answer yes-or-no autobiographical questions such as "Do you have any brothers?" by "modulating" their brain activity using either the motor imagery or spatial imagery task for affirming or negating.

In each condition the brain was scanned for distinct functional MRI (fMRI) activity in the supplementary motor area and the parahippocampal gyrus. The results revealed among the 54 patients 5 who could "willfully modulate" their brain activity according to the instruction. Four of the five patients were diagnosed as being in vegetative state and one as in minimally conscious state, all five due to severe traumatic brain injuries. In response to autobiographical questions the patient in vegetative state presented in five of six questions activity distinctive for either spatial or motor imagery task activation and indicating the right answers. The activation corresponding to the last question could not be decoded.

Another study additionally threw light on the condition of vegetative state. In order to gain greater knowledge in differential diagnosis between vegetative state and minimally conscious state, Di et al. (2007) evaluated the differences in brain activation in response to presentation of the patient's own name spoken by a familiar voice, in seven patients with vegetative state and four with minimally conscious state. Two patients in vegetative state failed to show any significant cerebral activation. Three patients in vegetative state demonstrated activation within the primary auditory cortex. The other two patients in vegetative state and all four patients in minimally conscious state not only demonstrated activation in primary but also in hierarchically higher order associative temporal areas. These two vegetative state patients showed clinical improvement to minimally conscious state observed three months later.

1.9 Late improvement from vegetative and minimally conscious state

The American Academy of Neurology (1989) and the Multi-Society Task Force on PVS (1994) consider vegetative state permanent if it lasts for 12 months or more after a traumatic injury, or 3 months after an anoxic injury. Despite a relative lack of scientific interest in these challenging neurological states (Laureys, 2006) there is growing number of single case and survey studies that suggest forgoing the use of the term "permanent vegetative state" altogether and to consider whether it supports a self-fulfilling-prophecy. This does not obviate the need for wider analysis.

Andrews (1993) presents a survey on recovery from vegetative state and the results of his own study on recovery of patients after four months or more in persistent vegetative states. In his study, 11 of 43 patients in vegetative state regained awareness. The rate of recovery in both his research and other studies unequivocally exceeds the error rate of 1.6 per cent estimated risk of prognostic error taken as a base for the definition of permanent vegetative state. Childs & Mercer (1996) report a single case of a young woman regaining awareness after three years. Heindl & Laub (1996) conducted a study exploring the difference of outcome after persistent vegetative state in 127 children and adolescents and found that 84% of the patients with traumatic brain injury and 55% with the hypoxic brain injury left persistent vegetative after 19 months follow up. Further studies on late recoveries are presented by Arts et al. (1985), Higashi et al. (1981), and Rosenberg et al. (1977).

A remarkable case is described by Voss et al. (2006): an extraordinary recovery of functional verbal communication and motor function in a patient who remained in minimally conscious state for 19 years.

The most remarkable finding in this study was the MRI assessment of transiently increased fractional anisotropy and directionality in the posterior midline cortices, interpreted as increased myelinated fiber densities and novel corticocortical sprouting, paralleling the emergence of the patient from minimally conscious state. The quantification of white matter reorganization shows long-distance rewiring in posterior medial cortices, possibly reflecting axonal sprouting or neurite outgrowth, maybe even related to neurogenesis which has already been reported in adult squirrel monkeys.

The prognosis of a person emerging from minimally conscious state or persistent vegetative state does not merely depend on the severity of disability. In addition to medical records and feedback from the patient, the interest and support of the caretaking system and especially of the family is crucial (Andrews, 1993; Reiss, 2004, p. 120).

1.10   Further investigations of consciousness

The investigation of consciousness is a major area of research with a very long history and with no common theory agreed upon as yet. Consciousness is an elusive phenomenon, too familiar to even think about having to define it, and indeed a non-circular definition of consciousness is hard to come by. Reductionist definitions and approaches in neuroscience can make it easier in certain circumstances to describe and assess states of consciousness but also tend to turn people into quantifiable objects and therefore treat – if not marginalize - them instead of relating to them!

As comatose and vegetative states are defined by the lack of awareness of oneself and the environment, in other words, absence of consciousness, it is fundamental to revisit the definitions and the assumptions they are based on and the concept of consciousness in itself including its cultural influences.

Although an in depth discussion of consciousness (see e.g. van Gulick, 2004; Güzeldere, 1995a) is beyond the scope of this paper, a short review of some features, current basic questions, alternative approaches and advanced theories of consciousness will help to explain the hypotheses of this research. It will become obvious how this reflection is far beyond just being an interesting academic philosophical discussion but demonstrates the essentials behind our everyday medical, ethical, social and humanitarian actions including decisions about support and life and death.

Questions and features of consciousness

One essential question might be if we look down the phylogenetic ladder from humans all the way down to amoebae, where are we to set the bounds of the "charmed circle" (Dennett, 1987, p. 161) to which only those who possess consciousness belong? Which animal, person or other cognitive system may be regarded as conscious and what states belong to it? Is consciousness an entity and should it be added to the list of fundamental elements of the universe like electromagnetic fields or gravity, or is it a property that an organism has? And if it is a property, is there a cut-off to demarcate the domain of consciousness from that of unconsciousness or non-consciousness or is it a continuum in between? How do we relate to the asymmetry between the mode of access to facts of one's own consciousness and the mode of access to facts about others' conscious states?

Because of its nature the first-person perspective is also often called the phenomenological approach, phenomenal consciousness or P-consciousness (Güzeldere, 1995b) and the third-person perspective is referred to as the physicalist approach, access consciousness or A-consciousness (Güzeldere, 1995b).

Furthermore Velmans (2002) calls into question the reductionist view of identifying consciousness primarily as a brain state. To supplement empirical scientific achievements, we could also open up to centuries of subjective research in consciousness, for example in Buddhist or other spiritual traditions and invite the possibility that in a deeper reality there is no "coherent thing" that is the "self" or "I" (Lancaster, 1997). This would give us new ideas for example about the binding problem in implicit and explicit processing and childhood amnesia (Lancaster, 1997) and about awareness in so-called unconscious states of coma.

Last but not least the mind-body problem and how awareness interacts with our body will need to be revisited. Most of these approaches coming from the field of philosophy will challenge the positivistic perspective of neuroscience but a comprehensive understanding of consciousness will likely require theories of many types.

A diversity of approaches that each in their way aim to explain the physical, neural, cognitive, functional, representational and higher-order aspects of consciousness is needed (van Gulick, 2004).

1.10.1 An integral theory of consciousness

In his "integral theory of consciousness" Ken Wilber (1997, 2001) did extensive data research among various types of developmental and evolutionary sequences which led to a "four quadrant" model of consciousness and its development: The "Upper Right" (UR) quadrant, the "Lower Right" (LR) quadrant, the "Upper Left" (UL) quadrant and the 'Lower Left' (LL) quadrant.

It is far beyond the scope of this paper to provide a complete summary of his theory; nevertheless introducing some of its features will offer a wider understanding and a broader framework for research in consciousness and therefore in comatose states.

Each of these quadrants includes both hierarchies and heterarchies. Each unit in a quadrant is what Koestler called a Holon, a whole that is simultaneously part of some other whole (like an atom is part of a molecule).

	INTERIOR	EXTERIOR
	Left Hand Paths	**Right Hand Paths**
	SUBJECTIVE	OBJECTIVE
INDIVIDUAL	truthfulness sincerity integrity trustworthiness	truth correspondence representation propositional
	I	**it**
	we	**it**
COLLECTIVE	justness cultural fit mutual understanding rightness	functional fit systems theory web structural-functionalism social systems mesh
	INTERSUBJECTIVE	**INTEROBJECTIVE**

Figure 2. The Four Quadrants and Validity Claims (Wilber, 1997)

The Four Quadrants and Validity Claims

The two "Right Hand" quadrants contain units, holons which all possess simple location: they can be seen with the senses or their extensions. They are all empirical phenomena ("Upper Right": atoms, molecules, etc. "Lower Right": galaxies, planets Gaia system, etc.). In other words they are objective ("Upper Right") and interobjective "Lower Right" realities. Both these quadrants can also be associated with third-person approach or access-consciousness.

The holons contained in the "Upper Left" quadrant represent a summary of the major evolutionary capacities of interior apprehension (sensation, perception, impulse, emotion, etc.) and can be associated with the first-person perspective or phenomenal consciousness.

The "Upper Left" represents the interior of a holon, whereas the Lower Left represents the collective form of individual consciousness, cultural or communal interiors, worldviews, or communally-shared sensitivity (magic, mythic, rational, centauric, etc.).

In the overall structure we have an upper half of quadrants referring to individual holons and the lower half to the collective forms. The left half refers to the interior or subjective forms; the right half to the exterior or objective aspects of holons. This creates a grid of exterior-individual (or behavioral, UR), interior-individual (or intentional, UL), exterior-collective (or social, LR), and interior-collective (or cultural, LL), or a grid of subjective, objective, intersubjective, and interobjective realities.

Each of the quadrants is described in a different type of language. The Right Hand quadrants representing objective realities are described in the language of "it", whereas the "Upper Left" represents first-person perspectives and is described in the language of "I" and the "Lower Left" expressing intersubjective realities is described in "we" language.

Furthermore Wilber postulates that each of these quadrants has a different "type of truth" or validity claim representing different types of knowledge and therefore different types of evidence and validation procedures. The most familiar validity claim is so-called objective truth (representational truth and the correspondence theory of truth) of the "Upper Right" quadrant. But it is not adequate to ask for objective truth if someone shares a feeling. The validity criterion in this situation is not truth, but truthfulness or sincerity. In the area of interobjective realities of the "Lower Right" quadrant the validity claim is functional fit explaining how individual holons fit and interact together in a system. In the "Lower Left" quadrant we are not focusing on the interaction of objects in physical space but how subjects fit together in cultural space. The question is for example: does my subjective consciousness fit with your subjective consciousness? The question is not simply whether it is true but whether it is good, right, appropriate, or just. The aim is not objective truth or subjective truthfulness but to come to a mutual understanding in a shared intersubjective space. The validity claim here is *appropriateness* or *justness* of our statements and actions which relates to ethics in the broadest sense (see below).

Each of the dozen theories of consciousness that Wilber researched contributes something very important, but partial. Consciousness is distributed across all four quadrants and each quadrant has correlates in all the others. Consciousness is anchored in the physical brain, but in the same way in interior intentionality. It is also not merely located in the physical organism but in cultural meaning and in the ecological system as well.

Chalmers' (1995) "easy problems" (such as cognitive integration in brain processes) can be understood by reductionist approaches of the "Upper Right" quadrant. But "the hard problem" (Chalmers, 1995), such as how physical processes in the brain give rise to subjective experience, remains an "explanatory gap". Wilber argues that this irreducible gap between matter and sensation cannot be bridged by physiology or any sort of reductionism from any quadrant to any other. It is just an aspect of the subject-object dualism which was clearly expressed by Descartes. Higher stages of consciousness disclose themselves only to postformal consciousness: in order to transcend this dualism the researcher needs to open up to transformation of consciousness in herself.

Wilber's conclusion is that there are "two wings of studying consciousness: the nonreductionistic 'simultracking' of all quadrants (behavioral, social, intentional and cultural) and the transformation of researchers themselves – which are both necessary for an integral approach to consciousness".

1.10.2 Altered states of consciousness

Chapter 1 of "Plum and Posner's Diagnosis of Stupor and Coma" begins with the topic of altered states of consciousness (ASC) Posner et al. (2007, p. 1) state that "normal consciousness depends on an intact brain, and that impaired consciousness signifies failure." But what is normal and what is non-normal or altered? What is the relationship between the two? What is our attitude towards ASC and how do we relate to them?

Charles T. Tart (1969, p. 1) who coined the term altered states of consciousness" (ASC) defines it as a state in which a given individual clearly feels a qualitative shift in her pattern of mental functioning. The person feels not just a quantitative shift, like being more or less alert, but also that some quality or qualities of her mental processes are different.

This contrasts with a normal or ordinary state of consciousness which is not something natural or given, but a highly complex construction or system of psychological structures and subsystems to interact with the physical, intrapersonal and interpersonal environment in accordance with biological and cultural conditions. Tart emphasizes that our ordinary state of consciousness is just a section in a continuum of consciousness which we define as normal from the background of our culture and therefore needs to be maintained by various subsystems to retain its identity and function. (Tart, 1983, p. 5, p. 63; 1972). It has adaptive value within a particular culture and environment; we benefit from this adaption and are also limited in our awareness and behavior in the same moment (Tart, 1969, p. 2; 1983, p. 33).

An ordinary state of consciousness requires an optimal range of exteroceptive stimulation; levels of stimulation either above or below this range appear conducive to the production of altered states of consciousness (Ludwig, 1969, p. 10).

Ludwig (1969, p. 18) also summarizes various functions of ASCs and describes adaptive and maladaptive expressions. The later includes attempts at resolution of emotional conflict, defensive functions in certain threatening situations conducive to the arousal of anxiety, breakthrough of forbidden impulses, escape from responsibilities and inner tensions, the symbolic acting-out of unconscious conflicts, the manifestation of organic lesions or neurophysiological disturbances and an inadvertent and potentially dangerous response to certain stimuli. Adaptive expressions include healing, avenues of new knowledge and experience, and social functions.

Cultures vary very widely in their appreciation of different kinds of altered states of consciousness. Eastern cultures for example offer many meditation practices and access to spiritual experiences. Some indigenous cultures believe that almost every normal adult has the ability to go into a trance state and be possessed by a god; the adult who cannot do this is psychologically handicapped.

Within our Western culture we have prevailing negative attitudes toward altered states of consciousness. We have a much better knowledge of psychopathological states than of positive or rewarding experiences (Tart, 1969, p. 2). Altered states of consciousness are not unfamiliar to us. We experience them for example when we get caught by strong affects like an outburst, when we give in to our addictions, when we experience sexual excitement, have strong dreams, go through deep meditation or drug experiences but also when we perceive pain, faint, die or enter a comatose state.

We fall into altered states of consciousness but we also yearn for them to disengage ourselves from our ordinary states of consciousness. Knowing our own altered states of consciousness is not only crucial for our personal development and health, it also reduces the anxiety of dying and it enables us to relate more deeply to people in altered states like dementia or coma (Tart, 1969, p. 2; Mindell, Amy, p. 35).

1.10.3 The dreambody concept

Another important philosophical topic which is far beyond the scope of this paper but also relevant to the question of consciousness and the possibility of contact and communication with people in comatose states is the mind-body problem. Due to limited space the concept will be briefly presented here, which is the basis of the method applied in this research.

In the early 1970s Arnold Mindell, a physicist and Jungian analyst discovered that dreams appear not only at night, but also during the day in the form of many experiences, including body symptoms; and that meaningfulness, on a personal but also collective level, can be found in the experience of symptoms as well as in dreams.

This mirroring of physical experiences in dreams Mindell (1985, 2004) called the *"dreambody"*. In order to understand this finding it is important to distinguish two different aspects of symptoms. Symptoms – as well as proprioceptive and kinesthetic signals in comatose patients – have an objective or consensus reality based aspect and a subjective or nonconsensus reality based aspect. The term "consensus reality" (CR) refers to the world of objectivity where you can measure, demonstrate and intersubjectively communicate about and agree on things such as symptoms, whereas the "nonconsensus reality" (NCR) aspect belongs to subjectivity where only you yourself have perceptions of your symptoms (such as proprioceptions, feelings or associations).

In other words symptoms can be described through third-person, access consciousness or "Upper Right" quadrant viewpoint, and through first-person, phenomenal consciousness or "Upper Left" quadrant perspective.

Like the unconscious in Jungian Psychology or the quantum wave function in physics the *dreambody* is a nonconsensus reality concept, a sentient, pre-signal experience which manifests in terms of dreams, slips of the tongue, unpredictable motions and also in body symptoms.

Due to the nonconsensus reality aspect, symptoms express not only personal but often also collective processes because human beings are also part of a bigger field which C. G. Jung called the collective unconsciousness (Mindell, Arnold, 1985, p. 13-20; 2000, p. 509-541).

Western health science has developed enormous knowledge of physiology and pathophysiology of the human body, invented sophisticated technical tools to diagnose and treat various medical conditions and offered many possibilities for positive change. In addition to the medical paradigm and its causal explanations Mindell proposes that symptoms always have an nonconsensus reality aspect and therefore are an expression of the dreaming, the background reality of our everyday experience. He also developed a detailed technology for tracking how experience manifests through multiple "channels", or modes of representation (Diamond & Jones, 2004a).

Exploring and unfolding the subjectivity of symptoms is a doorway to greater awareness, coherence, satisfaction and often also an improvement of symptoms (see also Weyermann, 2006). Having symptoms is not only distressing; from the nonconsensus reality viewpoint it is also means having important dreams and the chance of liberation and freedom from a rigid identity. As dreams looked at from the background of C. G. Jung's (1991, p. 158) theory of compensation, symptoms are also seen as a compensation for one-sided attitudes and therefore offer the potential for personal growth and well-being.

1.10.4 Summary and consequences of an integral approach to consciousness for relating to people in comatose states

The concept of consciousness is important and a deciding factor in diagnosis with practical and ethical consequences. If we do not perceive any expressive behavior in an unresponsive person, from the background of our limited and culturally influenced awareness, we cannot deny their consciousness: we can just admit that we do not reach this person.

Standardized assessment tools such as coma scoring systems or coma scales document the expressive behavior (access-consciousness) as that would be expected in ordinary states of consciousness. Event-related brain potentials and neuroimaging provide insights into the function and structure of the brain. These are objective, third-person (access-consciousness) and consensus reality based approaches to the question of consciousness but do not reveal any information about first-person (phenomenal consciousness) or non-consensus reality aspects.

Before we have reliable answers to these fundamental questions we have to assume that there is potential for consciousness in unresponsive patients. In following a one-sided and limited approach of measuring consciousness we run the danger of denying comatose patients' consciousness and marginalizing them. Setting a cut-off point for consciousness, for whatever reasons, is an arbitrary consensus. So far the evidence seems to be in favor of the potential for consciousness.

There is also evidence for consciousness in states where we usually presume that there is none. For example sleep and dreams are seen as merely non-pathological states of unconsciousness. However lucid dreaming had already been described in the West by Marquis d'Hervey de Saint-Denys at the end of the 19th century and in the 1990s researched by LaBerge (1990) and others.

In Buddhism and Hinduism there exist long traditions of practicing sleep and dream yoga which means practicing awareness during dreams and also during dreamless sleep stages (Varela, 2006; Chögyal Namkhai Norbu, 2002). The Bön Tradition in Buddhism goes back to the 9th century with monks practicing awareness in dreams and even in dreamless deep sleep stages to attain enlightenment.

There are no measurements to objectively assess nonconsensus reality experience or phenomenal-consciousness in unresponsive patients. As Wilber (1997) states, we cannot reduce intentional spaces [first-person experiences] to extensional spaces [third-person experiences] and then locate consciousness in a hierarchical network of physically extended emergents.

It is essential to extend our knowledge of physiology and neuroimaging data as correlates of consciousness and to extend our knowledge of medical treatment ("Upper Right"). People's reports from periods of unconsciousness ("Upper Left") represent another source of information about experiences in so-called unconscious states even though they may have a degree of uncertainty due to retrospectivity.

Furthermore Mindell (1999, p. 125) stresses the importance of exploring our own altered states of consciousness ("Upper Left") to become more familiar with them and as a prerequisite to relating to patients in altered states of consciousness, in order to reach out and to gain deeper mutual understanding (validity claim in "Lower Left") with people in comatose states and to not force them to relate to our ordinary state of consciousness.

Postulating states of unconsciousness (strictly speaking states without consciousness) may come from an aspect of our human nature, fear of the unknown, and from the deep need to establish and support the development of identity and diversity. The danger of saying that living people can be without consciousness however is that it supports a tendency of marginalization and a utilitarian ethic (Lanzerath, 1998), an ethic where privileges only fall to those who are able to look after themselves. In contrast, assuming consciousness as a continuum supports inclusivity and solidarity, and hence an ethic of care.

From that point of view coma is an extremely deep altered state of consciousness as Mindell proposes. This state differs radically from our ordinary state of consciousness but contains no barriers – besides/apart of a lack of personal experiences – which could prevent us from reaching out to them.

1.11 Rehabilitation methods for people in comatose states and vegetative states

1.11.1 Overview of rehabilitation methods

The Aspen Neurobehavioral Conference Workgroup on vegetative state and minimally conscious state (Giacino et al., 1997) proposed that interventions should be classified into one of two categories based on how essential each is to management. Basic interventions represent treatments that were regarded as essential to care and should be utilized across patients for whom they are appropriate such as range-of-motion exercises, positioning protocols, dietary parameters, and tone alteration methods. Optional interventions consist of treatment procedures that are considered nonessential but are appropriate for consideration on a case-by-case basis such as sensory stimulation procedures and pharmacologic trials.

The most widely used rehabilitation methods are (Nijenhuis & de Vetten, 2006):

2. Pharmacological interventions (including: L-dopamine, psycho-stimulants, anti-psychoplegics and opiate antagonists, hydrochloride naloxone)
3. Sensory stimulation (stimulating the reticular activating system [RAS] through stimulation of all five sensory pathways)
4. Physical treatment (passive range of movement, positioning protocols and hygiene management)
5. Hyperbaric oxygen therapy (inhalation of 100% oxygen inside a hyperbaric chamber)
6. Electrical treatment (deep brain stimulation [DBS] and median nerve stimulation)

These methods are usually summarized under the term coma stimulation or coma arousal therapy because they focus mainly on stimulating the reticular activating system through stimulation of one or all five sensory pathways and preventing environmental (sensory) deprivation.

The goal of music therapy (Aldrige et al., 1990; Gustorff, 1992; Herkenrath, 2006) is to develop methods of relating to and joining the patient's inner experience and situation, for example by following the tempo of the patient's pulse and rhythm of breathing. Zieger (1999) developed a method to enhance the possibility of dialogue with patients in coma and a system of translating overt behavior into potential messages.

1.11.2 Process-oriented Coma Work

Process-oriented Coma Work hereinafter referred to as Coma Work is a body of theory and practice for an awareness approach to patients in comatose, vegetative and other highly withdrawn states of consciousness.

Coma Work is an extension of Process-oriented Psychology developed by Arnold Mindell (1985, 2000) which is a multicultural, multileveled awareness practice including people (individuals, couples, families and large groups), and their natural environment.

Process-oriented Psychology, more commonly known as Process Work has roots in Jungian psychology, communication theory, Taoism and physics. Process Work emphasizes awareness rather than therapy, out of respect and trust in the wisdom and teleology of people's processes

Mindell assumes that the potential pattern for change and growth lies within the disturbing process itself. Even disturbing events such as dreams, physical symptoms, addictions, family and relationship problems, group conflicts and social tensions reveal an inner order and coherence that can bring new information vital for our personal or collective growth when all the information, within our awareness and on the verge of it, gets unfolded with curiosity and respect.

In working with people in comatose states Coma Work accepts the medical paradigm and its understanding of pathology but follows a non-judgmental, phenomenological description of processes.

Coma Work is based upon a set of **assumptions** (Mindell A., 1989, p. 5; Mindell, A., 1999, p. 34, 277) which are partially examined in this study. Mindell states that people in comatose states are not unconscious but in an extremely deep altered state of consciousness in which the person is not relating to ordinary reality. Processes within the altered states of consciousness are meaningful and seeking for awareness and completion; they are up to that moment the unknown parts of our wholeness and individuation process.

Minimal signals such as eye movements (also under closed eyelids), facial microexpressions, changes in skin color, vocalizations, and changes in breathing rhythm often interpreted as reflex behavior in the medical paradigm are seen as potentially meaningful and as expressions of inner processes.

This perspective reflects the dreambody concept. By means of special communication methods these signals can be used to relate to comatose patients. Mindell assumes that people in coma are potentially able to perceive themselves and their environment.

Mindell (1999) also mentions various **goals** in Process-oriented Coma Work. In contrast to most coma arousal therapies the goal is not to awaken or heal people primarily although this sometimes happens, but to make contact, to communicate with the comatose person and in advanced stages even to establish a binary system of communication.

It is essential to encourage comatose people to believe in their experiences and to perceive themselves and their environment. Coma Work aims to orientate the person to their situation, provide a sense of loving companionship, support social participation and enable them to participate in making decisions.

The foundation for applying Coma Work methods is an **attitude** of believing in the comatose patient's capacity to perceive and relate to outer and inner experience. Even in the midst of a medically and personally difficult situation the comatose person is seen as a human being following a process. In order to facilitate the comatose person's process the coma worker needs a deep trust in nature, an openness to the unknown and an appreciation of all states of consciousness and conditions of life. Since it is not the primary goal to arouse and awaken but to support, accompany and follow them it is ethically important to be open to follow them towards more alertness and recovery or journeying towards death.

In addition to these assumptions and attitudes a wide range of **meta-skills or feeling qualities** (Mindell, Amy; 1995) permeating every approach help to support the comatose person's experiences. Among other meta-skills sensitivity, curiosity, openness, welcoming experiences, compassion and love for example deeply influence the effects of interventions.

Coma Work covers on the one hand **methods** which are easy to learn and can be applied by relatives and friends of the patient, and on the other hand more advanced and complex ones to be used by trained facilitators.

The most direct and effective way to make contact, build up communication and accompany the comatose person is to support and join their altered state of consciousness and relate to minimal signals. The coma worker notices all minimal signals and frames them verbally back to the patient in an atmosphere of appreciation and deep respect to support the emerging process in the nonverbal communication. This kind of framing is the most basic way of amplifying signals.

To start with, especially in acute and very withdrawn stages, joining the patient's breathing is a very basic intervention which helps the facilitator to join the patient more closely. Speaking in the rhythm of the patient's breathing, during the exhalation phase, helps to tune into their experience. It slow things down, allows time for the comatose patient to follow and maybe to react, and time for the coma worker to notice subtle feedback.

Noticing the channels or modes of representation in which the signals arise, helps to choose the interventions according to the patient's process. Naming experiences and framing them by using verbs corresponding to the channels in which they occur, supports the patient in experiencing these processes more intensely.

Amplifying movement or proprioceptive signals is one of the main interventions. Amplifying movement signals can be done by either carefully completing or sometimes also slightly resisting them. Proprioceptive signals such as relaxation can be amplified for example by naming them, additionally by pacing the intonation of the framing according to the quality of relaxation or adding sounds mirroring the quality of relaxation. Noticing and reporting back to the patient even the tiniest positive feedback with a welcoming attitude helps to unfold the emerging process (more examples of interventions see also chapter 2.4 and Mindell, Amy; 1999).

1.12   An integral approach to people in comatose states

The invention of the positive pressure mechanical ventilator in the 1950s, the subsequent development of intensive care and enormous improvements in medicine radically increased the survival rate of critically ill patients. People who would have died years ago survive and regain consciousness today; others die, stay in coma for weeks and recover or transfer into vegetative state, minimally conscious state or other remote states of consciousness. The question of consciousness in comatose patients is one of many in this context and touches on essential medical, psychological, philosophical, spiritual and especially ethical aspects. The conundrum is not only how we get to know if unresponsive people have awareness but also how we relate to the range of consciousness and related experiences within ourselves and how this relationship is influenced by culture and correspondingly how far people's comatose states are also influenced by the social and physical environment.

Extensive research has been done from an "Upper Right" quadrant approach. As Wilber proposes, research in consciousness [and therefore in coma] requires nonreductionistic simultracking of all quadrants and the transformation of researchers themselves. Mindell's Process Work and its application in coma offer a down-to-earth method including a personal, relationship, field or collective and environmental approach.

1.12.1 Coma as an experience on a personal level

What is different about working with comatose patients as distinct from other critically ill patients is the lack of normal verbal communication, interaction and feedback. Not being able to reach someone throws us back on ourselves and often reveals our lack of contact to ourselves. Who is at home?

The ability to make contact with people in comatose states is strongly influenced by our attitudes towards life and death and how we relate to our own altered states of consciousness (Mindell, 1999, p. 35; Sakamoto, 2004). The more we know ourselves and our own altered states of consciousness and are interested in them, the more comfortable we feel during contact with people in comatose states.

The characteristics of altered states of consciousness mentioned above such as the clear qualitative shift in mental functioning, alteration of thinking, loss of control, to name just a few, make us avoid them most of the time. Our attitude towards suffering or no longer being able to meet culturally highly valued qualities such as achievement makes us uncomfortable. Not knowing or believing that there is a potential for consciousness in comatose people may keep us mute; on the other hand it supports a lack of contact and isolation on both sides. We speak to babies and look for reactions and feel into the atmosphere. Why not with comatose children or adults? Furthermore Mindell (1999, p. 124) identifies central edges, or temporary limits of our identity, in learning Coma Work:

- Shyness about and awkwardness in assisting someone who is in an altered state of consciousness
- Fear about one's own altered state of consciousness
- Fear of death
- Inhibition about being expressive with sound, touch, and movement
- Fear and shyness about intimacy and contact

In addition to these attitudes the range of his skills influences the Coma Worker's experience. Every single effort of a caregiver applying loving attention will support a comatose person. In addition some fundamental skills will deepen the work and change the personal experience of contact with a comatose person.

A basic skill is to be able to hold an inner observer or meta-communicator where one is aware of what is happening in the relationship with the comatose patient, within oneself and in the atmosphere, being able to reflect processes happening in the moment and being able to frame them in a welcoming way where it this needed. This requires openness to the unknown and fluidity in shifting from consensus reality to non-consensus reality, from ordinary to altered states of consciousness.

The Coma Worker's capacity for intimacy will help to create more closeness and will help to amplify proprioceptive or kinesthetic processes through touching the person where it is appropriate. The Coma Worker's ability to express feelings and atmospheres in words or sounds and his ability to amplify the comatose person's movements will deepen the work.

The Coma Worker's experience, attitudes and skills strongly influence his experience of the relationship.

1.12.2 Coma as an experience in relationship

Coma is not only a private experience of the person in this state but also an experience in relationship. Having looked at some intrapersonal aspects of this relationship in the caregiver it is worthwhile to study also some inter-personal facets. Watzlawick's well-known statement "one cannot *not* communicate" is no less relevant in a relationship with a comatose person. We can even notice more communication happening where there is less awareness. As we know from Watzlawick's communication theory and as expounded in Process Work, we do communicate verbally but also nonverbally. Process Work studies the process, the flow of signals, not only in language but in various channels or modes of representation. Four basic channels of perception are described: auditory, visual, movement and proprioceptive. In addition to these sensory perceptions taste and smell may also be relevant in some cases. Furthermore Process Work formulates two composite channels: the relationship and world channels, which encompass experiences communicated or noticed in relationship to someone, or to collective, global, social, or political events or institutions (Diamond & Jones, 2004a; Mindell, 1987).

Signals and communication which are closer to our identity are called primary; processes further away from our identity are called secondary and often emerge in so-called double-signals. These signals do not go along with the intention and awareness of the owner but reveal marginalized, repressed or even totally unknown, new and emerging processes. Both the caregiver and the comatose person are communicating with more or less awareness.

In this way all our personal and internalized collective assumptions and attitudes about the comatose person, the altered state the person is in and about the relationship, will be communicated by various signals and influence the atmosphere. For example a pure medical attitude assuming all experiences and reactions of the patient as pathological, may have negative effects and possibly contribute to deepening the comatose state (Mindell, 1989, p. 92; Mindell, 1999, p. 261), whereas a loving interest, an appreciation of simple being and deep compassion may show positive effects.

Relationships with caregivers, partners and the whole family system may play another important role in the process of the comatose person. In addition to medical records and feedback from the patient, the interest and support of the caretaking system and especially of the family is crucial to the outcome (Andrews, 1993; Reiss, 2004, p. 120). Reiss also describes how coma may amplify pre-existing personal and relationship issues; working on these can have positive effects as well (2004, pp. 109). From a family system theory point of view dynamics happening in the family sometimes mirror the patient's processes.

Contact and communication may also be influenced by the experience and the extent of awareness of both partners. A parallel to this is seen in Sogyal Rinpoche's (1993) accounts of people's dying processes. Quite often people die in pain and agony and sometimes, having practiced awareness over decades and maybe accompanied by an experienced spiritual teacher, die more peacefully and enter deep spiritual experiences. However awareness may be hindered or more difficult due to analgo-sedation or psychoactive drugs. The balance between motives for sedation and for the possibility of gaining more awareness needs to be well considered. Both may serve to support the comatose person's process.

1.12.3 Coma as an environmental, collective and field experience

The intensive care unit offers an environment in which to save people lives; without it most of the critically ill patients would die. The atmosphere is characterized by acute urgency and high strain, by high tech equipment focusing on objective measurements and their control. Hannich (2009) did a survey study on psychosomatic and psychosocial aspects of ICUs where he elaborates which physical, social and psychological strains patients and also staff are exposed to. Hannich has brought together studies on various stress factors in the physical environment of intensive care units. Many of these environmental conditions aggravate altered states of consciousness (Ludwig, 1969, p. 10); for example, overstimulation by repeated medical treatments, interventions, constant, sometimes very loud noise but also lack of stimulation of various senses are characteristic. Hannich also explores social and psychological stress factors and explains how these stress factors often lead to detachment or withdrawal in the staff (by denial, escape into activity, objectification, and decrease of contact). An enormously high incidence of postoperative delirium varying in various studies up to 73.5% is also caused partially by environmental factors (van der Mast, 1999, Osterbrink et al., 2004).

These phenomena arise not only due to limited space and finances but are also an expression of cultural values. We favor consensus reality over non-consensus reality, effort over rest, rationality over emotionality and so on. We gain collective support when we have intense proprioceptive processes perceived as symptoms but we easily become marginalized by having intense emotional processes dismissed as mental disorders. As studies on reports from patient's experiences during periods of unconsciousness (Lawrence, 1995) have revealed, people fear being stigmatized as a result of sharing memories which fail to meet expected consensus reality ideas.

All these cultural values and belief systems create a "we", a kind of cultural identity, and at the same marginalize other experiences. These attitudes may be more or less conscious but constitute a field within our culture, in intensive care units and in the context of comatose states. All these positions can also be seen as roles in society or in a group of people but they are also inherent in us.

1.13 Deduction of hypotheses

The object of this research was to test Process-oriented Coma Work interventions and the assumptions they are based on. Mindell (1989) assumes that coma is not a state of absence of consciousness as it is still defined in neuroscience (Posner et al., 2007) but an extremely deep altered state of consciousness in which there is potential for awareness, the ability to hear and therefore a possibility for contact and communication. According to Mindell the deciding factor is the nature of contact. Unrelated approaches such as asking people everyday questions or demanding of them to respond to given instructions, such as in the Glasgow Coma Scale, will not result in strong effects in comatose people and therefore classify them as comatose. A critical aspect and essential prerequisite is a radically related contact by a person who believes in the meaningfulness of the comatose person's experiences and who relates to their state of consciousness and to the minimal signals the person is communicating by. Such attitudes and skills will enable the facilitator to reach out, establish contact and get feedback.

Operationalizing consciousness in comatose persons from a third-person perspective in overt behavior such as kinesthetic and proprioceptive signals is not only challenging but also still difficult due to a lack of standardized assessment tools. Comatose persons who are additionally analgo-sedated are also less likely to demonstrate such reactions. Therefore the feedback of the sympathetic nervous system activity expressed in electrodermal activity (dependant variable) as a kind of covert behavior and precursor of overt behavior (Zieger & Hildebrandt, 1996) was used to assess awareness in comatose people and the effectiveness of Process-oriented Coma Work interventions.

Directive alternative hypotheses

1. Process-oriented Coma Work interventions (independent variable: related contact) will lead to an increase in the tonic aspect of skin conductivity (SCL)

    a) compared to values measured in the baseline

    b) compared to values measured during Glasgow Coma Scale assessment (independent variable: unrelated contact)

2. Process-oriented Coma Work interventions (independent variable: related contact) will lead to an increase in the phasic aspect of skin conductivity (SCR)

    a) compared to values measured in the baseline

    b) compared to values measured during Glasgow Coma Scale assessment (independent variable: unrelated contact)

2.   METHODS

2.1   Sample

2.1.1   Selective criteria

Comatose patients with GCS value <8 were included in the study whereas comatose patients medicated with catecholamine, with artificially reduced temperature, using a pacemaker or not understanding the German language were not admitted.

2.1.2   Sample description

The study was conducted between August 2008 and May 2009 in the neurological intensive care unit of a hospital for psychiatry and neurology. The study was approved by the ethics committee of the Medical Association of Düsseldorf. Informed consent was obtained from each patient's legal surrogate.

Originally 16 comatose patients were admitted to the study. Due to various reasons such as medical emergency interventions, patients' transfer to other wards, awakening from coma, dying and organizational or technical problems the sample reduced to 7 patients (4 female and 3 male). Due to a small number of patients fulfilling the criteria and being available on the ward also people in very deep comatose states additionally ventilated and analgo-sedated had to be included as in many other studies as well. As assessed by a neurologist Glasgow Coma Scale score varied from 3 to 7 (M 4.4, SD 1.6). Age varied from 64 to 88 years (M 76.3, SD 7.4). Sex and age were registered but not evaluated within the study. Six patients were intubated and analgo-sedated with Dormicum™, Fentanyl™ or Propofol™. One patient was medicated with Keppra™. Patients' diagnoses covered amongst others: subarachnoid hemorrhage, stroke, brain stem incarceration.

Due to the limited access to comatose patients no control group existed. Instead the assessment of coma depth was used as a control condition representing an unrelated kind of contact versus the highly related contact in the experimental situation.

Table 4. Description of the sample group

Patient	Sex m/f	Age	Ventilated & analgo-sed.	GCS scores E+M+V	4.4 (1.6)GCS score total
1	f	64	x	2+1+1	4
2	m	80	x	1+1+1	3
3	m	72	x	1+1+1	3
4	f	75	x	1+1+1	3
5	m	77	x	1+1+4	6
6	f	78	x	1+1+3	5
7	f	88	-	1+1+5	7
Min./Max		64/88			3/7
M (SD)		76.3 (7.4)			4.4 (1.6)

(m=male, f=female, E=eye response, M=motor response, V=verbal response)

2.2 Assessment of coma

The depth of coma was assessed by means of the Glasgow Coma Scale (Teasdale & Jennett, 1974). The scale has a good sensitivity and reliability (intraclass correlation coefficient, $r\text{-}p=0.8$ to 1 for trained users [Prasad K., 1996]), is easy to perform and the procedure takes about five minutes. As already described in chapter 1.2.2 the scale comprises three tests: eye, verbal and motor responses. The neurologist greeted the patient and asked questions to test for verbal response and the level of orientation. Further he asked the patient to open her eyes and to move maybe a hand. If the patient after repeated instructions was not verbally responding at all the neurologist used painful stimuli such as pressing into the nail bed of fingers or rubbing the breastbone to test for responses.

This test is used for assessment of coma depth and at the same time in this research design as value of the independent variable (quality of contact). The procedure of the Glasgow Coma Scale represents an unrelated contact.

2.3 Recording of electrodermal activity

The physiological data were recorded with a physiological-medical instrument (PARPORT-R™[1996], PAR Medizintechnik GmbH, Berlin, Germany). This instrument allows recording of maximum six channels. Off-line recordings were carried out by means of electrodermal activity (EDA). Skin conductance was measured by applying a constant voltage to the two electrodes (bipolar measurement with constant 0.48 V). The PARORT-R device split the EDA signals into tonic (SCL) and phasic (SCR) changes. Skin conductance level was measured in integer values of micro Siemens. The measuring range of skin conductance response extended from 0 to 0.1 μS/cm2. Data were recorded each second. Two standard silver-silver chloride (Ag/AgCl) disk electrodes (10mm diameter) filled with iso-tonic electrode paste were attached to the skin with appropriate-sized double-sided adhesive collars on the hypothenar and thenar eminence of the non-dominant palm (Boucsein, 1988).

2.4 Process-oriented Coma Work interventions

Since Process-oriented Coma Work is characterized by radically relating to the comatose patient's process there is no fixed protocol or program of Coma Work interventions to follow. Nevertheless there are some basic steps and frequently used interventions which can be described especially with people in extreme deep altered of consciousness. At the beginning a trained Coma Worker will join the patient's breath as far as possible. He will breathe loudly so that the patient can hear his breath and by that indirectly also getting more in contact with his own breathing. Joining the patient's breathing also helps the Coma Worker to feel into the patient and the atmosphere. The Coma Worker will speak in the rhythm of the breathing and will introduce himself and share his intentions. Further on the Coma Worker would verbally encourage the patient to deeply trust and follow her inner experiences. The Coma Worker may also express the atmosphere in between them or in the room. After a few minutes, and in the rhythm of the breath and speaking on the exhalation, the Coma Worker tells the person that he will touch her wrist (if it is medically appropriate). The worker will then gently touch the patient's wrist and will slightly press the wrist as the person inhales, releasing the pressure on the exhale. Signals, channel of experiences or the atmosphere are named and expressed out of a quality of appreciation, wonder and welcoming in order to unfold processes. Kinesthetic signals such as subtle movements of a finger will be amplified by simply naming the movement and also maybe carefully helping to complete the movement or sometimes by carefully resisting the movement and supporting a movement dialogue. Qualities can also be expressed by sounds. The patient might be invited to follow her images, thoughts, feelings etc. according to her process and the channel she is experiencing in the moment. Every intervention is aimed to pick up and to support and unfold experiences which are on the way to happening. The Coma Worker looks attentively for feedback to his interventions. All changes such as a deepening of the breath, a swallowing or sudden movements but also pauses or breaks in activity are seen as positive feedback and again are named and encouraged. Lack of reactions or no change of dynamic are seen as negative feedback and a cue to change interventions, follow another track or sometimes have a break (see also Mindell, 1999).

2.5   Videotape recording

Recording was done by means of digital video camcorder (Canon MV400), focused on the patient's face to document any auditory, visible proprioceptive or movement signals.

2.6   Procedure

After informed consent obtained from each patient's legal surrogate the experimental situation began by sticking the electrodes onto the patient's non-dominant hand. After a few minutes when the stuff was informed to not disturb during the five minute baseline, the recording was started to record the following periods for 256 seconds as for the following stages. Nobody was present in the patient's room during the baseline measurement. After this first step a neurologist led through the Glasgow Coma Scale. A minimum of 30 minutes of rest was incorporated in order to ease potential reactions from testing with painful stimuli. In the next step it was planned to assess responses to familiar contact of relatives or close friends compared to an unrelated contact during the Glasgow Coma Scale assessment and to a non-familiar but clearly related contact from a trained Coma Worker. This experimental condition could not be realized due to lack of relatives. Finally contact with and interventions by a Coma Worker followed for 30 minutes as presented in the chart below. The measurements were always taken in the 22nd minute for 256 seconds.

Table 5.   Research procedure

Baseline		Glasgow Coma Scale assessment 5 min.		Break mini-mum 30 Min.	Contact of relatives		Break min-mum 30 min.	Intervention Coma worker 30 min.	
SCL	SCR	SCL	SCR	-	SCL	SCR	-	SCL	SCR
256 seconds from the beginning		256 seconds from the beginning			256 seconds starting in minute 22			256 seconds starting in minute 22	

(SCL=skin conductance level, SCR=skin conductance response)

Table 6.   Revised research procedure

Baseline		Glasgow Coma Scale assessment 5 min.		Break mini-mum 30 Min.	Intervention Coma worker 30 min.	
SCL	SCR	SCL	SCR	-	SCL	SCR
256 seconds from the beginning		256 seconds from the beginning			256 seconds starting in minute 22	

(SCL=skin conductance level, SCR=skin conductance response)

In patient 1, 2 and 6 electrodermal activity measurements during the Glasgow Coma Scale could not be included into the analysis due to either technical problems or the neurologist who could not conduct the GCS within the required time setting.

Patients were accommodated in one- or two-bed rooms, so disturbance from other patients and their care could not be completely avoided. Interventions were conducted in the afternoon between 1 and 5 p.m. In order to reduce movement artifacts (Ebbecke-waves) in electrodermal activity measurements the hand with the electrodes should not be moved or touched. The room temperature was constant during the stages.

2.7 Data analysis

First the data was descriptively analyzed in an explorative data analysis. Lilliefors test for normality and graphical methods were used to test if the data was well-modeled by a normal distribution. If the data set was fulfilling these requirements a t-test for matched sample was lead through. If they are not normally distributed a non-parametric Wilcoxon signed-rank test for two related samples was applied. The raw data was analyzed with a graphical method for artifacts.

The statistical processing of the data was carried out with the statistical software package SPSS Statistics 18.0 for Windows.

3.   RESULTS

3.1   Results of normality testing

The exploration of data for the skin conductance level (SCL) variable revealed an acute peak (kurtosis: 7.0), and right-skewed curve (skewness: 2.645). Lilliefors' test for normality distribution mirrors this result (p=.0) for rejecting the null hypothesis of normal distribution. Graphical methods such as the histogram and Q-Q plots confirmed this result.

The exploration of data for the skin conductance response (SCR) variable revealed a lower, wider peak (kurtosis: -2.30), and left-skewed curve (skewness: -0.34). Lilliefors' test for normality distribution revealed a non-significant result (p=0.20) for rejecting the null hypothesis of normal distribution. The histogram and Q-Q plots for normal distribution show only a few outliers not severely violating the requirements for normal distribution. Bortz et al. (2008) even argue that biometric variables can be assumed to be normally distributed. Due to this controversy and especially the small number of the sample a normality distribution was not assumed for the time being and a non-parametric analysis was made.

The descriptive statistics for the 7 patients are presented in Table 7. Great differences in mean and median are marked bold. In order to not lend too much weight to the extreme values, the median of the raw data was used for values in skin conductance level and response in the analysis with the non-parametric Wilcoxon signed-rank test for two related samples.

3.2 Skin conductance level and skin conductance response values in baseline, GCS and Process-oriented Coma Work intervention

The descriptive statistics for the 7 comatose patients are presented in Table 7; mean and median values of the raw data of all patients in the three experimental conditions.

The tonic level of skin conductivity (SCL) of comatose patients shows nearly no variation in the baseline (from 0.0 to 0.41 μ S/cm2) (M 0.0, SD 0.0). The mean of median raw data increased during Glasgow Coma Scale assessment (M 0.75; SD 0.50) and even further during the Process-oriented Coma Work intervention (M 2.0; SD 2.0).

The phasic aspect of skin conductivity (SCR) varied from 15.91 to 44.16 in mean and from 13 to 44 in median μ/100 S/cm2 (M 30.64, SD 12.21) in the baseline. The mean of median raw data increased during Glasgow Coma Scale assessment (M 37.25; SD 11.76) and again even further during the Process-oriented Coma Work intervention (M 53.0; SD 15.58).

Table 7. Patients' skin conductance level and skin conductance response values in baseline, GCS and Process-oriented Coma Work intervention phase

Patient	GCS	Baseline		GCS		Intervention	
		SCL	SCR	SCL	SCR	SCL	SCR
		M (Mdn)	M (Mdn)	M (Mdn)	M (Mdn)	M (Mdn)	M (Mdn)
		μS/cm2	μ/100 S/ cm2	μS/cm2	μ/100 S/ cm2	μS/cm2	μ/100 S/ cm2
1	4	0 (0)	36.63 (36)	-	-	1.00 (1)	51.80 (52)
2	3	0 (0)	44.16 (44)	-	-	6.00 (6)	85.66 (86)
3	3	0 (0)	22.15 (22)	1 (1)	25.02 (24)	3.00 (3)	55.92 (56)
4	3	0.004 (0)	41.99 (41)	0.85 (1)	52.89 (51)	1.00 (1)	45.47 (45)
5	6	0.41	15.91 (13)	1 (1)	36.13 (32)	1.00 (1)	44.46 (39)
6	5	0 (0)	40.59 (39)	-	-	1.96 (2)	56.58 (44)
7	7	0 (0)	20.04 (19,5)	0 (0)	41,74 (42)	0.00 (0)	49.11 (49)
Min./ Max		0/0 (0/0)	15.91/ 44.16 (13/44)	0/1 (0/1)	25.02/ 52.89 (24/51)	0/6 (0/6)	41.46/ 85.66 (39/86)
M (SD)		0.06 (0.15)	31.64 (11.84)	0.71 (0.48)	38.94 (11.61)	1,25 (1.26)	55.57 (14.07)
M (SD) of Mdn raw data		0 (0)	30,64 (12.21)	0.75 (0.50)	37.25 (11.76)	2.00 (2.00)	53.00 (15.58)

(P=patient, GCS= Glasgow Coma Scale, SCL=skin conductance level, SCR=skin conductance, M=mean, Mdn=median, SD=standard deviation)

3.3 Effects of Process-oriented Coma Work intervention measured in skin conductance level

Measurements of the tonic aspect of the skin conductivity (SCL) revealed a significant increase and result for the effectiveness of Process-oriented Coma Work interventions with people in comatose states (p=0.013; Z=-2.23) compared to the baseline measurements. The results confirm the first hypothesis (1a). In a similar way also the second hypothesis (1b) is confirmed. The contact during the Glasgow Coma Scale assessment showed also a significant increase of SCL (p=0.042; Z=-1.73) but the Process-oriented Coma Work interventions presented a higher significance compared to the baseline (p=0.013) than the unrelated contact during the GCS assessment. No significant difference could be measured between GCS assessment and Process-oriented intervention.

Table 8. Effects of Process-oriented Coma Work intervention measured in skin conductance level (SCL)[b]

	SCL increase in GCS condition compared to BL	SCL increase in IV condition compared to GCS	SCL increase in IV condition compared to BL
Z	-1.73a	-1.000a	-2.23a
Asymptotic signify-cance (one-sided)	.042	.16	.013

(SCL=skin conductance level, BL=baseline, GCS= Glasgow Coma Scale, IV=intervention, Z=z-score, a=based on negative ranks, b=Wilcoxon test)

Figures 3 to 5 demonstrate the increase of the tonic aspects of skin conductivity (SCL) in 256-second epochs in patient 3 from the baseline (Mdn 0 μS/cm2) to Glasgow Coma Scale assessment (Mdn 1 μS/cm2) and to Process-oriented Coma Work intervention (Mdn 3 μS/cm2).

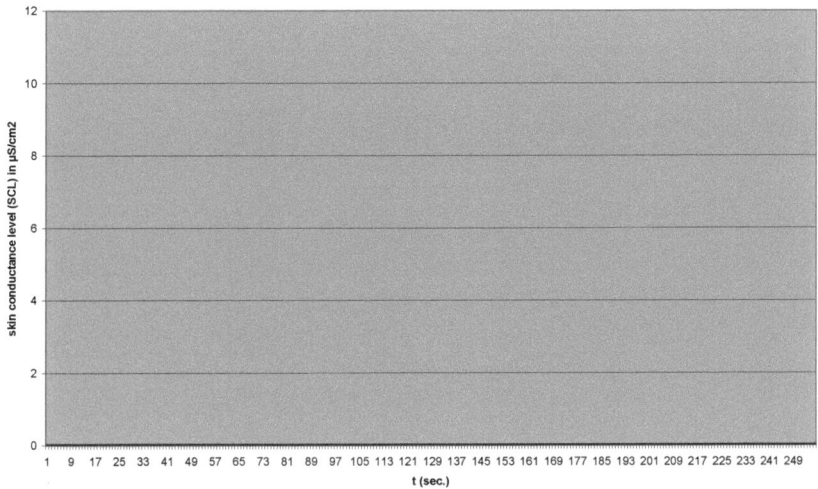

Figure 3. Skin conductance level (SCL) of patient 3 during baseline phase

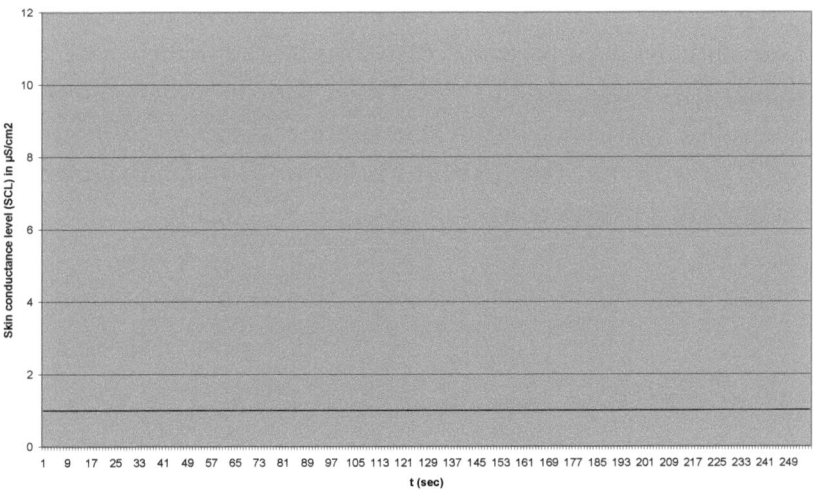

Figure 4. Skin conductance level (SCL) of patient 3 during GCS assessment phase

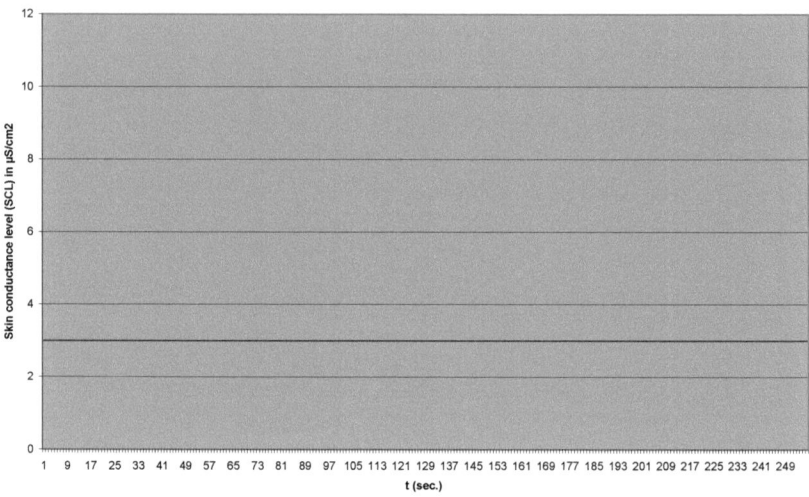

Figure 5. Skin conductance level (SCL) of patient 3 during Process-oriented Coma Work intervention phase

Measurements of patient 3 demonstrate the tendency of grad-ual increase of skin conductivity. Other patients skin conductivity show subtle variations within the baseline (patient 5 in Figure 6), the Glasgow Coma Scale (patient 4 in Figure 7) and in the interven-tion (patient 2 in Figure 8).

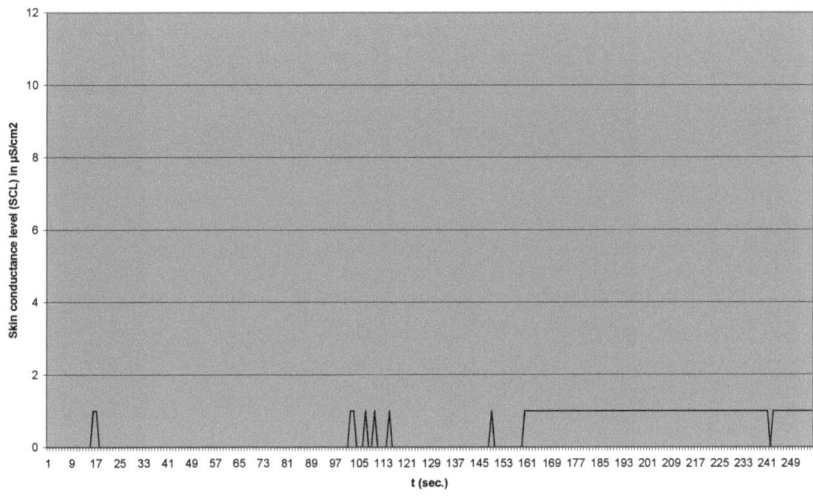

Figure 6. Skin conductance level (SCL) of patient 5 during baseline phase

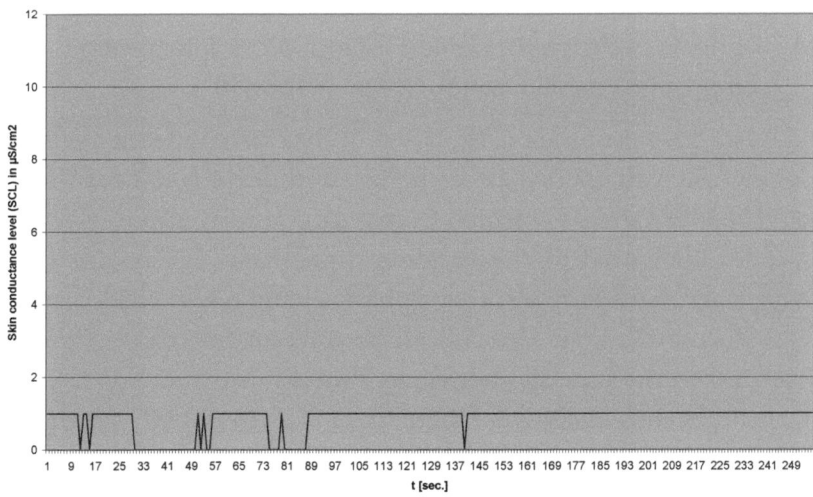

Figure 7. Skin conductance level (SCL) of patient 4 during GCS assessment phase

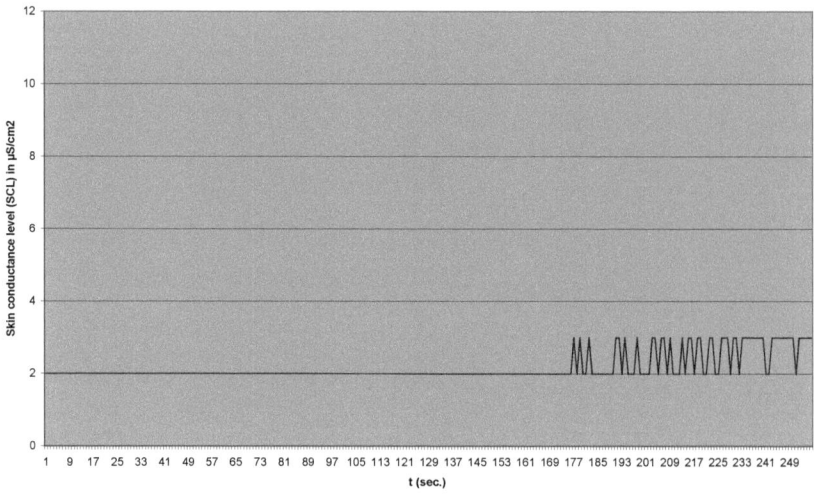

Figure 8. Skin conductance level (SCL) of patient 2 during Process-oriented Coma Work intervention phase

3.4 Effects of Process-oriented Coma Work intervention measured in skin conductance response

Measurements of the phasic aspect of the skin conductivity (SCR) of comatose patients revealed a highly significant result for the effectiveness of Process-oriented Coma Work intervention (p=0.009; Z=-2.37) compared to the baseline (hypothesis 2a). As for tonic changes in electrodermal activity, phasic changes also yielded an increase during Glasgow Coma Scale assessment (p=0.034; Z=-1.83) compared to the baseline but again Process-oriented Coma Work intervention showed a higher increase of SCR (p=0.009). From that point also the fourth and final hypothesis could be confirmed (hypothesis 2b).

Table 9. Effects of Process-oriented Coma Work intervention measured in skin conductance response (SCR)[b]

	SCR increase in GCS condition compared to BL	SCR increase in IV condition compared to GCS	SCR increase in IV condition compared to BL
Z	-1.83 a	-1.47a	-2.37
Asymptotic signify-cance (one-sided)	.034	.071	.009

(SCR=skin conductance response, BL=baseline, GCS= Glasgow Coma Scale, IV=intervention, Z=z-score, a=based on negative ranks, b=Wilcoxon test)

Figures 9 to 11 document the increase of the phasic aspect of skin conductivity (SCR) in 256-second epochs in patient 3 from the baseline (Mdn 22 μ/100 S/cm2) to Glasgow Coma Scale assessment (Mdn 24 μ/100 S/cm2) and to Process-oriented Coma Work intervention (Mdn 56 μ/100 S/cm2).

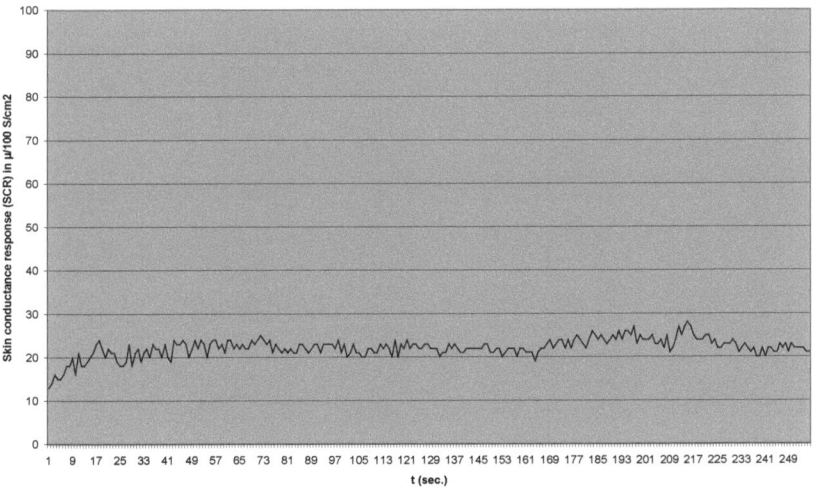

Figure 9. Skin conductance response of patient 3 during baseline phase

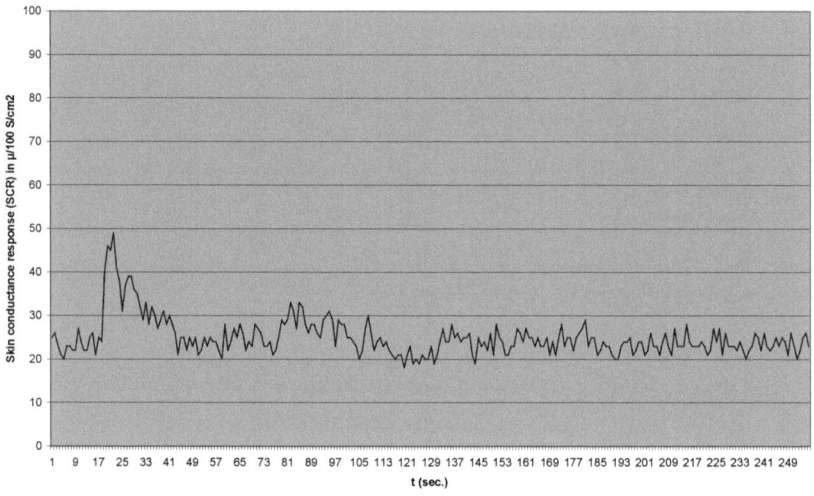

Figure 10. Skin conductance response of patient 3 during GCS assessment phase

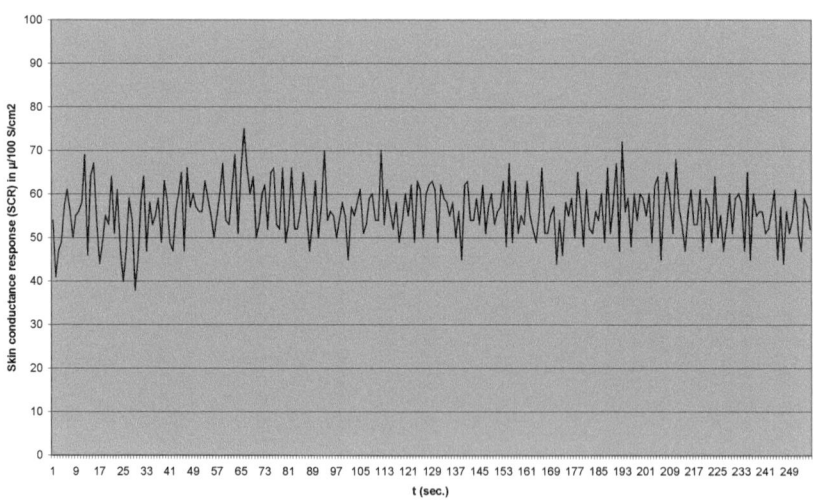

Figure 11. Skin conductance response of patient 3 during Process-oriented Coma Work intervention phase

4.   Discussion

In this chapter the results of the four hypotheses of this research will be discussed. Subsequently limitations and weaknesses of this study will be discussed in detail.

4.1   Comatose patients' ability to hear

The significant increase of skin conductance level and the highly significant increase of skin conductance response during Process-oriented Coma Work intervention reveal further evidence for comatose patients' ability to hear. Yagi & Baba (1983), Guerit et al. (1999) and Kane et al. (2000) showed similar results in comatose patients and Kotchoubey et al. (2002), Owen et al. (2006) and Di et al. (2007) for patients in vegetative states. Recent studies using fMRI (Schiff et al., 2005; Owen et al., 2006) revealed evidence for activation of associative cortices in vegetative patients which signifies awareness in non-responsive patients. Inferring awareness and high cortical processes from increased electrodermal activity expressing sympathetic nervous system activity is more difficult. Naqvi & Bechara (2006) and Tranel & Damasio (1994) argued that higher brain areas are not necessary for reflex SCRs to non-emotional, but they are necessary for SCRs in response to stimuli that have acquired emotional value. Greater increase in electrodermal activity during Process-oriented Coma Work intervention compared to contact with a neurologist during the Glasgow Coma Scale assessment which is louder and more invasive suggests further evidence for not only reflex behaviour but higher cortical processes in comatose patients.

4.2 Awareness in comatose patients

The effect of increasing skin conductance level and response indicate at least minimal awareness in comatose people and a process of increasing vigilance. Hildebrandt et al. (1998) identified increased sympathetic nervous system activity and reintegration of the sympathovagal balance as the process of emerging from coma. In their study this dynamic was expressed in changes of heart variability, skin conductance level and skin conductance response. The significant increase of electrodermal activity in response to Process-oriented Coma Work interventions represents a covert behavior which precedes overt behavior.

Skin conductance responses are also seen as one of the most reliable indicators for an orienting response which is a response to novel events that are not aversive (Vossel & Zimmer, 1998).

4.3 Effects of radically related contact

From the significant and highly significant increases in electrodermal activity in response to Process-oriented Coma Work intervention we can infer that a radically related approach to comatose patients is a key factor. The Coma Worker's ability to join the comatose patient by entering the altered state of consciousness, believing in the reality of the patient and being able to pick up and amplify minimal signals play a major role. These skills and also the attitudes and meta-skills discussed in chapter 1.7.2 strongly support processes in the relationship between the patient and the facilitator and therefore also affects the state of consciousness of the patient. Consciousness cannot only be ascribed to an individual as if he were a separate entity. Consciousness is within the individual, in the relationship and in the field (Mindell, 2000). In other words: consciousness is distributed in all quadrants: is subjective, objective, intersubjective and interobjective (Wilber, 1997).

Radically relating to the comatose patient's process supports what is happening in the patient in the moment. Precisely amplifying and unfolding what is happening in the comatose patient has greater effect on the sympathetic autonomic nervous system than strong or even painful stimuli.

4.4   Defining and assessing consciousness

Although these results should be interpreted carefully, when they are taken together with other results discussed in this paper there is increasing evidence for the suggestion that comatose patients cannot be diagnosed as unconscious in the sense that they are not perceiving themselves and their environment. The present definition of consciousness in neuroscience does not disclose its arbitrary and culturally influenced stance. When we do not admit our own limitations in awareness and communication skills we tend to underestimate the comatose patient's consciousness. We do not admit that we do not know how to reach out to this person but instead we diagnose them by the absence of our expectations. This attitude tends to support marginalization and a utilitarian ethic. In contrast, assuming that consciousness is a continuum supports inclusivity and solidarity.

4.5   Limitations

Several limitations have to be considered when interpreting the data. The generalizability of the results is limited by the small sample size. The research would need a larger number of patients therefore needing an appropriate intensive care unit or access to several wards admitted by the ethics committee. Access to comatose patients who are not analgo-sedated is quite rare.

Another limitation of the interpretation of the results is the fact that six out of seven patients were not only in coma but in addition analgo-sedated. Their reactions can be presumed to be reduced. It can be assumed that the reactions and the increase of sympathetic nervous system activity would have been more intense in nonanalgo-sedated patients such as was the case with one patient who could not be included in the sample. This patient (GCS score: 4) demonstrated increasing activity during the intervention and finally at the end of the intervention woke up and gazed directly at the Coma Worker for about 6 minutes. Beyond this it is unclear how analgo-sedation influences the lack of reactions but also the kind of reactions. However patients reacted to the intervention even though they were in coma or under analgo-sedation.

Research with comatose patients would also need an instrument which is more sensitive in the very low range of the channel for skin conductance level to also allow for the differences of patients' sympathetic activity in very low value, close to zero. The lack of variance in patients' skin conductance level (SCL) in the baseline (Table 7) is probably due to this relatively insensitive measurement.

The analgo-sedated patients were also intubated. The Glasgow Coma Scale was used to assess the depth of coma because this scoring system is well known, including in this ward, easy to perform and mostly also used in similar studies. But as already discussed in chapter 1.2.2 the Glasgow Coma Scale is not suitable for use in intubated patients (Hinder et al. 2001). Alternatively the Full Outline of UnResponsiveness (FOUR) (Wijdicks et al., 2005), a new scoring system designed to potentially replace the GCS, could be used instead but the staff would have to be trained.

Another important issue to be mentioned is the lack of a control group and the variations in experimental conditions. From a methodological point of view a matched control group would be needed for a systematic analysis. Besides ethical objections it would result in a far bigger project than this format allows. Alternatively a variation of the sequence of the second condition (GCS) and the third condition (Process-oriented Coma Work intervention) could be used. On the other hand if Process-oriented Coma Work intervention were to have a strong effect, patients might no longer be in the same stage of coma after the intervention. A more realistic alternative experimental condition could be established by inventing an unrelated non-painful contact of the same duration as the Process-oriented Coma Work intervention to reveal differences in the nature of contact as a basic prerequisite.

A matched control group with an unrelated intervention of the same duration would also ensure that the Glasgow Coma Scale assessment does not influence the increase in electrodermal activity during the intervention.

5. CONCLUSIONS

These first results of and experiences in this exploratory research should be carefully interpreted but nevertheless are promising and prompt further research directions. The results also represent first evidence of validity for Process-oriented Coma Work intervention as an effective rehabilitation method for comatose patients.

The importance of Process-oriented Coma Work lies not only in its positive effects of relating and communicating with comatose patients and in further contributions to rehabilitation processes but also in the paradigm shift involved.

Assuming comatose states as extremely deep altered states of consciousness will not only lead to a new definition of consciousness and doorways to relating to seemingly lost people but also to a deeper connection to ourselves and to our social and physical environment and promote deeply ethically motivated behavior. Admitting comatose states as extremely deep altered states implies a continuum of consciousness where I am not separated from the comatose person and where it is not only his problem but also a challenge to the relationship and the whole system involved. This implies inclusivity and an ethic of care. Comatose patients challenge us to extend our awareness, to reflect on our ethical values and belief systems, to appreciate all states of consciousness, to value people for their pure existence and not because of their achievement, an attitude which leads to compassion.

The effectiveness of Process-oriented Coma Work interventions in relating to comatose patients would help to reduce one of the most oppressive problems for their relatives and caretakers of comatose patients: the lack of familiar communication and relatedness. These results provide evidence that comatose patients do perceive and react even when they do not show, or only show very minimal overt behavior. This could encourage people to not give up and also trust more their own experience of contact and relationship. These methods are learnable by everyone and could help caregivers to support the patient. The importance of the support system and how it influences even the prognosis is already discussed in chapter 1.8.2 (Andrews, 1993; Reiss, 2004, p. 120).

Believing in comatose patients' awareness and supporting them in trusting their experiences in these states could facilitate subsequent processing of these experiences and reduce the high incidence of delirium (Van der Mast, 1999) during intensive care and posttraumatic stress disorders after coma (Schelling et al., 1998).

Process-oriented Coma Work interventions could also contribute to reducing the documented extent of up to 43% of misdiagnosis in vegetative states (Andrews, 1996; Schnakers et al., 2009).

6. RECOMMENDATIONS

The question of awareness in patients in so-called unconscious states could also be explored in patients in vegetative states. It would slightly shift the focus but would give more control to experimental conditions than in an intensive care unit setting. Comatose people in an intensive care unit are in an emergency situation. Their medical situation often changes quickly and drastically so the control of experimental conditions is very difficult. Alternatively, a study including only comatose patients without analgo-sedation would allow the testing of Process-oriented Coma Work interventions. Comatose patients without analgo-sedation will show greater responses, overt behavior and maybe even first-person accounts of consciousness.

In a larger project with more resources a research design including control samples would increase the internal validity of the results. Since placebo or non-treatment conditions would not be suitable a comparison with an established coma stimulation approach such as sensory stimulation could be relevant. A further approach would be to vary the amount and intensity of related contact. In such a control group comatose patients could be accompanied by untrained person who is instructed to talk to the comatose patients and to also gentle touch the person. The latter condition would reveal the effects of joining the patient's state of consciousness and the amplification and interaction with the patient's minimal signals. This kind of design requires more therapists and a greater number of patients but would allow a process-outcome analysis and reduce the allegiance effect.

Documentation of the mode of ventilation, especially the aspects of spontaneous breathing rhythm and volume would not only help to distinguish potential influences and artifacts on electrodermal activity but could serve as a further dependent variable. Spontaneous breathing is also strongly influenced by sympathetic activity and is a result of reintegration of sympathovagal balance. An increase of spontaneous breathing was observed during Process-oriented Coma Work intervention in this research. It is also a crucial issue in the often challenging weaning process.

Exploring possible effects of touching the patients' skin during the intervention would increase the reliability of the results in electrodermal activity. Alternatively touch could be controlled or parallelized in the matched control group.

Use of a coma depth assessment tool which is suitable for intubated patients such as the Full Outline of UnResponsiveness (FOUR) scoring system would be required. Tools for standardized documentation of kinesthetic and proprioceptive signals such as the Facial Action Coding System (Ekman & Friesen, 1976) which focuses only on the face would be needed to also document overt behavior.

In whatever kind of institution or clinic the research is conducted, extensive presence of and close cooperation with all professionals on the ward will be crucial and will facilitate the whole project

APPENDIX I: SINGLE CASE TRANSCRIPT

Translated verbatim transcription of a session

This is a transcript from a session with a comatose man which could not be included in the study. At this stage of the study the effect of Process-oriented interventions should have been measured by the increase of the sympathetic nervous system activity expressed in the heart rate variability (dependant variable) as a kind of covert behavior and precursor of overt behavior (Zieger & Hildebrandt, 1996). The heart rate variability describes changes of the time interval between individual heart beats (interbeat interval, IBI). The variation in interbeat intervals, as the electrodermal activity, is strongly influenced by the autonomic nervous system. Hildebrandt (1998, 1999) describes wakening from coma in neurophysiological terms as a successive increase of the sympathetic activity of the autonomic nervous system and a re-establishing of the sympathovagal balance. Unfortunately it turned out that the local monitor Infinity SC 7000 interface only allowed an output of heart rate every two seconds. In consequence the heart variability could not be evaluated from this data. Since this case was one of a few patients who were comatose but without ventilation and analgo-sedation and clearly showing strong effects of Process-oriented Coma Work interventions it is described in this appendix. The session was videotaped with a digital video camcorder and afterwards a translated verbatim transcription of the session was made. The amplification of signals could have been more precise but the meta-skills expressed and interventions as a whole contributed to the awakening from the comatose state of this patient for the first time after being in coma for several days.

This patient was a man aged 54 with the following diagnosis: apoplexy (embolism right A. cerebri med., cerebri ant., cerebri post. and Aa. Cerebelli), Korsakoff's syndrome, hemi-spastic on left side, spasmodic hiccup and multidrug-resistant Staphylococcus aureus (MRSA). Assessment with the Glasgow Coma Scale carried out by a neurologist revealed a score of 4 points (eye response: 2, motor response: 1, verbal response: 1). He was not intubated but had a nasal stomach tube. Due to the infection with MRSA he was isolated in a single-bed room and special clothes had to be worn by the staff.

Baseline phase:

The procedure was the same as already described in the research design. During the 256 seconds recorded baseline the patient was lying in his bed with his head turned slightly to the right. His breathing was regular and slow. His eyes were closed. He groaned a few times and showed chewing and swallowing motions. Nothing noticeable happened. His heart rate varied between 73 and 99 beats per minute (M 82.9, SD 42.5).

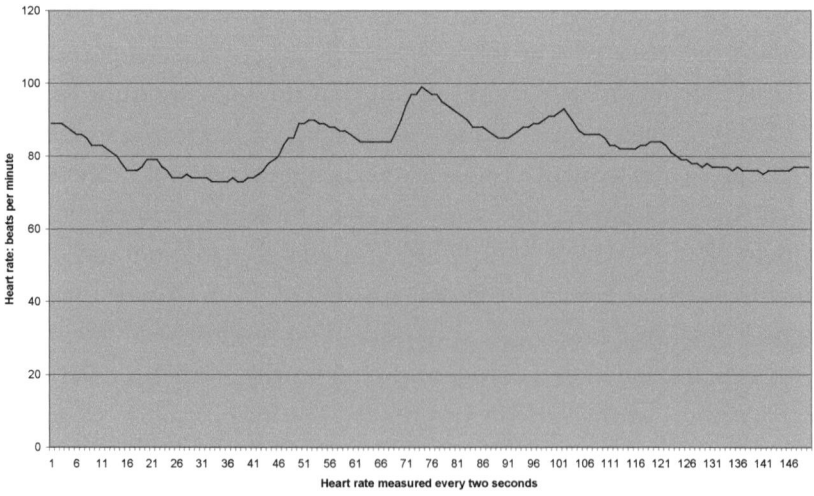

Figure 12. Heart rate single case patient during baseline phase (256 seconds)

Glasgow Coma Scale phase:

In the Glasgow Coma Scale phase while a neurologist assessed the state of consciousness the patient showed several times spasmodic hiccups, coughed once, slightly (2mm) opened his eyes after painful stimuli but overall he did not show much reaction. His heart rate ranged between 84 and 94, on a slightly higher level than in the baseline (M 87.9, SD 1.95). The heart rate was quite irregular and oscillating.

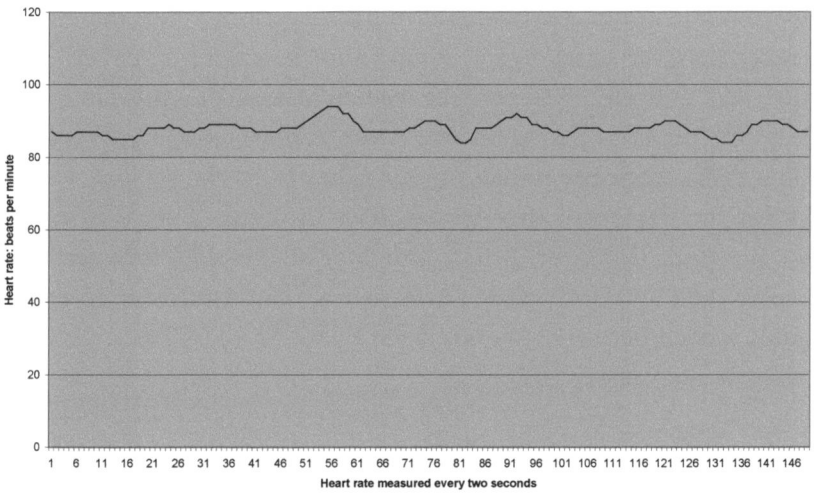

Figure 13. Heart rate single case patient during GCS assessment phase (256 seconds)

Process-oriented Coma Work intervention phase

The observed 256 seconds sequence of the intervention phase should have started in min. 37:27. That was postponed because a surgeon came for a surgical consultation and interrupted the interaction. The verbatim transcription of this sequence started at min. 39:27.

Short summary follows of what happened before the beginning of the transcription. In the first 21 minutes more movements appeared and grew stronger in his right arm, upper body and head.

He started to open his eyes very slightly. He was holding the Coma Worker's thumb. There followed more eye movements under closed eyelids. His right foot started to move. He was grinding his teeth. He showed tension in his right arm and jaw muscles. Tension and intensity were evident. His temporomandibular joints were crepitating. He was squeezing the Coma Worker's hand. He strongly flexed his right arm.

Minimal signals increased constantly, grew stronger and more intense. When the Coma Worker announced that he was leaving the patient made a strong movement in his direction. Upon the request to receive a clear signal to stay longer another strong signal emerged which was interpreted as positive feedback. A short while later (min. 53:05) the patient opened his eyes wide and focussed clearly on the Coma Worker for the remaining six minutes of the session. He did this for the first time after several days in coma. The next session took place the day after. A few days later he could be transferred to an early rehabilitation ward. The heart rate during this intervention session varied between 76 and 95 (M 85.97, SD 3.644).

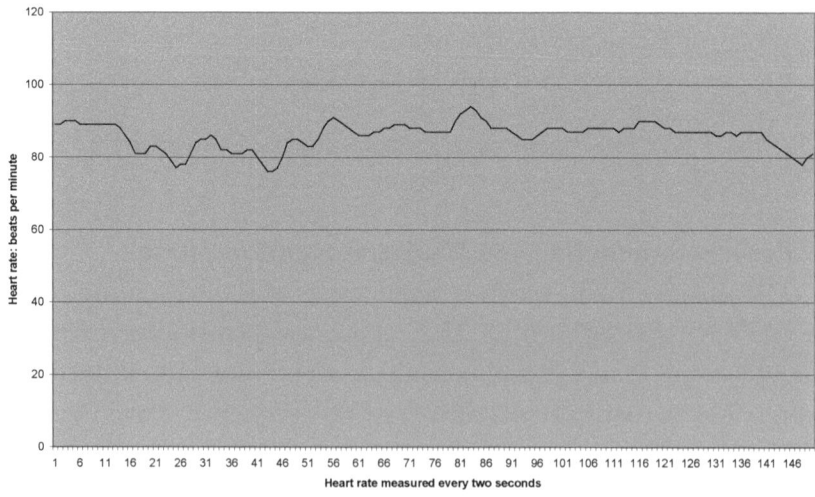

Figure 14. Heart rate single case during Process-oriented Coma Work intervention phase (256 seconds)

The measurements of the heart rate did not show a direction or difference in these three phases and in the awakening from coma. Hildebrandt et al.'s study (1998) also revealed that heart rate is not a significant parameter for distinguishing different coma depths whereas heart rate variability as an integrated parameter is significant.

Baseline phase:

Min.:	Behavior of the patient:	
00:00	Eyes closed, breathing slowly, mouth slightly open, head turned slightly to the right. Noise from outside of the room, nurses working, alarm signal, bleep from other patients' monitors next door.	
01:18	Coughing up, and swallowing	
01.18 01:53	Chewing motions, eyes constantly closed.	
02:04	Coughing, swallowing, eyes opened 2 mm for a very short moment	
02:30 02:36	chewing	

02:54	Brief groaning	
03:03	Yawning, mouth opening widely, eyes very briefly slightly open	
03:17	Brief groaning	
	(various noises from other rooms in the ward)	
05:00	End of baseline phase	

Glasgow Coma Scale assessment phase:

Neurologist is assessing the state of consciousness by using a GCS scale.

Min.:	Behavior of the patient:	Behavior of the physician:
09:46	Eyes closed, breathing slowly, mouth slightly open, head still turned slightly to the right.	
10:02		Physician is entering the room
10:15		Mr. Meyer (a pseudonym), hallo! (he is speaking in a loud voice!)

10:21		Please open your eyes
10:24	Hiccups	
10:28	Hiccups	Mr. Meyer, my name is Dr. X. I'd like to look into your eyes (he is also touching his chest). Could you please open your eyes?
10:44		(he is tapping on the patient's left cheek, several times) Mr Meyer!
10:57	Afterwards Mr. Meyer opened his eyes slightly.	I want to see what he does when I open his eyes (the physician opens patient's eyes with his fingers. Patient is not closing them actively.
11:08	Patient opens 2 mm the eyes for a brief moment.	Mr. Meyer could you open your eyes wide! Mr. Meyer. Can you understand me? Mr. Meyer can you understand me?
11:22		(Physician testing the flexibility of the patient's right arm)

11:28		(Tapping his face again, several times to get any reaction.)
11:35		(Physician speaks to the assistant): absolutely, opening eyes only after forced verbal approach, 2 points! Verbal responses none. I will try once more, asking him to talk.
11:44		Calling wouldn't have been enough.
11:45		No verbal response. Motoric reaction: I shall try by calling him.
11:52	Hiccups!	Mr. Meyer, I am squeezing your hand, please do it to me. Could you please do it as well!?
12:04	Chewing.	Nothing! Even though it is his better hand. On the other side he has a hemiplegia.
12:15	Spontaneous movement in his upper body	Just now he has spontaneous movement. But not on command.

12:26	Hiccups	(the physician lifts the patient's right arm and tests the patient to hold the arm up on its own.) We'll see if he holds up the arm. It is additionally difficult because he has ...
12:30	Groaning. Very slight opening of eyes.	Additionally he has a fracture here, an old one. It is an uncompleted healing.
12:38	Groaning a bit more strongly and making noises.	(Continues moving his right arm) He can not hold it on his own.
12:50		(Physician to assistant): Spontaneous movement, no! Physician: no grimacing! I try it on the other side (left arm).
12:55		Now I am testing a painful stimulus (testing pain stimulus, on the nail of one finger of the right arm).

13:16	Eyes open slightly, hiccups.	Mr. Meyer! (very loud, after painful stimulus) Now the eyes are open for a moment. Inner side is more painful than the outer side. No grimacing!
13:38		I do it on the other side, too. What also should be painful is rubbing the sternum.
	Eyes open slightly	I have the impression that he becomes a bit more restless but motorically he
	Hiccups Eyes slightly opened for a second	doesn't really. Maybe the legs. Maybe spontaneous movement.
14:12	Coughing He opens his eyes again very slightly.	(nurse coming in and speaks to the physician)
14:22		Difficult to say. Spontaneous movements, yes. Reactions nearly none, I would say. What would you say (to the assistant)?
	Hiccups and slightly opened eyes	(Assistant): maybe 2 points.

14:49	Hiccups	It will hurt one more time, Mr. Meyer! I am doing that quite strongly. It should hurt. Nothing besides a kind of restlessness which I perceive.
15:00	**End of Glasgow Coma Scale assessment phase**	

Process-oriented Coma Work intervention phase

The detailed verbatim transcription starting from 22nd minute was postponed for 2 minutes to the 24th minute (time: 39:27) due to an examination by surgeon.

Min.:	Behavior of the patient:	Behavior of the physician:
39:27		… What you sense? Mm-mmh.
	Mouth starts to open, eyes (under closed eyelids) move faster	What you see? Yes, what do you see! Trust all that what you see!
	Big, strong movement of the upper body to the right! groaning	Yes! Mmmh, yes.

39:54	Movement of head, lips, groaning, movement of the mouth. Coughing and opening eyes wider, audibly grinding teeth!	Notice what you see! Yes. Trust your images! Right. Look at it, see what you see. Yes, trust your images! Yes, look precisely at it! Wow.
40:20	Movement of lips and coughing. Chewing movements and upper body movements to the right	Yes, looking and intensity in these pictures, in your experiences. Perceive what you experience.
40:56	Bigger movement in the upper body.	Look at it, as on a big screen. Figures, colours, landscape, places. Yes. Shapes, mmh.
41:47	Coughing	Trust what you experience, what you see.
42:06	Lips smacking brows moving, eyelids, eyes, corners of his mouth are moving	Yes, intensity is important, the power. I see your eyebrows moving, lids, corner of the mouth. Mmh, yes!
42:46	Head movement to the right	Trust what you are experiencing!

43:19		You are hearing inside --- sounds --- voices --- tones!
43:44	Mouth opens slowly. Snoring a bit. Stronger upper body movement, chewing motions	Feel what you are feeling --- your body --- emotions And if you are tired, it is also fine. Sleeping is fine too, dreaming is good too.
	End of heart rate recording (256 seconds) at 44:42	
44:40	Head and upper body movements clearly to the right!!	I will lay down your arm carefully and will visit you again tomorrow.
45:06	Strong coughing!!	Yes ... unless it is important to stay longer then it would be good to get a clear signal from you. O.K. of course I stay a bit longer. mmmh
45:39		O.K., I am fine to stay a bit longer.
45:45	Coughing	Yes, that was a strong cough!

46:09	Holding my thumb and my hand.	Yes, I feel that you are holding my thumb the whole time and gripping my hand. Mmmh, yes.
46:28	Right leg moves	Yes, moving your left leg.... No right leg! (Breathing with him and making sounds.)
47:40		I'll put my hand onto your chest carefully. Yes, I am wearing gloves. (making sounds according to the breath)
48:10	More movements of the upper part of the body	Yes, (breathing). Yes!!! I see the movement in your chest and in your legs. Yes! I am following the move-ments in your legs, yes. O.K.
49:58		Yes, follow what you are experiencing. Yes, that is the best guide. Mmmh, yes.

50:25	Upper part of the body movement, head movement to the right.	I want to take my hand carefully off your chest and then I will put it on your forehead.
50:36	Making sounds with his mouth and chewing movements. Subtle head movement to the left and right. Chewing movements and swallowing.	(Putting my hand on his forehead). (Stroking his forehead)
51:16		Yes, I see how your right arm is moving from side to side.
51:44 52:28	Coughing and chewing Swallowing, making sounds!! Coughing, groaning, sounds – eyes start to open.	Yes, great. Good swallowing. Trust the experience you just had. (I am repeating the sounds). Oh!! Mmmmh …. Trust your body (making sounds with him)
52:41	Eyes opening wide!!!! Coughing! Groaning.	Yes, I see your eyes opening! Yes!!

53:05	Eyes opening very big and focussing on me!! MORE OR LESS UNTIL THE END OF THIS SESSION FOR THE NEXT 8 MINUTES!!!	Hi, Hi, yes, wow! Wow! I see your eyes big and open! Yeah, hi! Wow! See what you see! Trust your body. (making sounds with him together)
53:57	Sounds, still focussing with open eyes, coughing. Chewing, groaning, (a nurse comes in)	What an exciting journey. I see your open eyes and how you look at me. Yes, Hello Mr. Meyer. Wooooow! We are getting visitors again. Yes, I look a bit strange, strangely dressed up (due to MRSA infection). But it is necessary at least at this time. Yeah! Wow. Welcome! The most important is that you are trusting what you are perceiving. Your whole life, every moment. If not it is O.K. too. And your body …. Wow, yes. …..

55:55	Still looking, hiccups, ... Chewing, hiccups.	Trusting ourselves is one of our greatest gifts. Not what others think or say about us but what you think, feel and perceive about you. Great to see you. You are in charge of things. (Stroking his forehead, amplifying sounds with him)
56:58	Making sounds	Feel your diaphragm … feel your belly.
57:12	Hiccupping (he looks very present and awake)	O.K. …. You are here in a hospital in an ICU and the physician who had examined your belly was a bit insensitive! He has examined your stomach and intestines. Feel what you are feeling.
58:12	He is watching with big eyes meanwhile. He has continuous hiccups. (Alarm bleeps)	Let any images come up. What images comes to you? Follow your fantasy. If you were to see someone with hiccups. What is the first fantasy? What comes to your mind?

59:20		Yes, let everything out. Everything that has to come out! Let it out. (Amplifying sounds)
	Hiccups.	Wow, great. (To the nurse) You are needed. It is bleeping ... I am taking my hand off your belly. Hallo Mr. Meyer (Nurse): Hallo Mr Meyer O.K. that was exciting Mr. Meyer. Trusting yourself. Trusting what you perceive. I see how you look at me, great! Welcome. I am putting your arm slowly back on the bedcover and will see you again tomorrow.
	End of the session	

Appendix II: Personal Experiences and Reflections

Introduction

The writing of this diploma thesis marks a milestone on my professional and also personal path. The journey on this path would not have happened without all the people who supported, helped, accompanied, loved, but also challenged me by criticizing me or arguing with me on the way and without nature encompassing and connecting all of us and giving me the drive to move forward especially in challenging periods. From that point of view this project and the associated explorative empirical research is a huge co-creation and collaboration described from my personal perspective.

In sharing some personal experiences, developments and motivations I am adding a counterpart and complement to the empirical approach of deducing from the general to the specific. My experiences, the processing of them and the learning steps arising from them give some insight from within and in addition hopefully will reveal some typical (psycho)dynamics and roles in the field of coma and altered states of consciousness.

Origins, planning and preparatory work

First ideas and motivations for this project date from 2001. I remember that the impetus to research coma came from my interest in deep internal states, my own introverted side, the potential importance of experiences in comatose and other altered states of consciousness, the ability to communicate with people in coma, my background in craniosacral therapy - a sensitive approach to body work - and finally my personal experiences with my first wife and my mother going through these states. Later on I became even more aware of how much this work is connected to my own nature and process.

Having already had some experience in Process Work and also in craniosacral therapy which developed my skills in noticing subtle signals and various states of consciousness, I started to study and train in Process-oriented Coma Work and to research the topic of coma in neuroscience. My vision was to undertake research for my studies in psychology at university and in Process Work and in through that research bridge neuroscience, psychology, psychotherapy and philosophy. My aim was also to demonstrate for the first time in an explorative empirical study what Arny and Amy Mindell and colleagues have been discovering and already practicing for more than twenty years around the world; that people in coma are not in a state of unconsciousness but in an extremely deep altered state of consciousness, that we can communicate with them and that a key factor is a radical way of relating to them. This purpose, its realization on an intensive care unit where the biomedical model is most pronounced, and my chosen framework of an empirical research study in the realm of non-consensus reality led to many challenges and constellated various growing edges in me.

I remember one of my supervisors drawing my attention to the potential difficulties of my research design in assuming a direct connection between a non-consensus reality intervention and a measurable outcome in consensus reality as a kind of efficacy study. He also pointed out the potential consequences of very ambitious projects such as an extended period of personal and professional struggle. I could not fully pick up his recommendations at that time. A part of me was still siding too much with and submitting myself to the empirical model, the acceptance of hard facts, marginalization of subjective perceptions and relationship, and finally also with having to do the research on my own. Doing research exploring the potential and meaningfulness of subjective experiences in coma and focusing on measurable outcomes as results was partially a polarization but also an unconscious identification at the same time.

Apart from doing exciting research I was also unconsciously caught in a power struggle, fighting the inner and outer attitude of marginalizing inner worlds by trying to use the same empirical means. The realization that this dynamic was at work took a long time and in consequence resulted in significant loss of energy. From early on, issues of marginalization of inner experiences, various altered states of consciousness, ambition, isolation, feeling stuck and power dynamics, including feelings of hopelessness as an aspect of it, were part of my personal process which on another level also are connected to the topic of coma and vegetative states.

My enthusiasm and ambition were huge but my hesitations and doubts in facing such a pioneering project as a beginner in a new and unfamiliar professional field, where the role of a psychologist or student of psychology does not belong and being more or less on my own, were not much smaller. So getting trained in Process-oriented Coma Work, investigating the topic in the academic field of neuroscience, developing a research design and getting ready for the first step out in the world and searching for a suitable intensive care unit took me a long time.

Finding a clinic in which to conduct my research and making contact with psychologists and physicians ushered in another phase of this project. I began to understand how coma and vegetative states are not exclusively an experience of the person concerned but also an experience in the relationship with caretakers and in the collective.

When I met with psychologists or physicians and shared the assumptions of Process Work, the specific approach to comatose people and my research design I was often offered suggestions such as to give standardized instructions to comatose people and measure the physiological parameters. Usually it required considerable effort to explain the essence of engaging with and radically relating to someone in a coma by relating to the state of consciousness the person is in and to the experience the person is having by noticing, following and amplifying her minimal signals. The difficulties and negative replies or refusals I was confronted with in the search for an intensive care unit where I could conduct my research made me aware how much I am also touching a collective ground. After I finally found an intensive care unit in a university clinic and I met the head of the department, it took nine months of phone calls and emails to finally hear that they would not have suitable patients for this research.

I remember well this meeting where I presented my proposal for this research. In his busy day he took time for me and was interested, especially when I showed a brochure of a conference about altered states of consciousness on the intensive care unit, which I had attended. When I left I was wondering about my low mood. I needed some time to realize that I must have faded out other signals indicating negative feedback to my request.

Probably I could have shortened this time of waiting and trying for another nine months if I had been able to not only hear the "yes" but also to notice the "no" in the double signals in that moment. It would have been even more helpful and constructive if I had already been aware that all the issues, belief systems and edges around coma, altered states of consciousness and how we do not only relate or not relate to people in coma but also to our own altered states of consciousness and what holds us back or even scares us, would be present in the moment while talking with him about my research project.

Facilitating these parts in him, in me and as roles in our society might have led to an intense and deep meeting and even potentially to the start of the project. I myself needed more awareness to realize that my project had already started even though it was not running in the way I had envisaged. These collective dimensions were not so much my focus at that time and not part of my proposal. So I had to wake up to this dimension and to recognize for example that I am also in a role of a troublemaker questioning some basic medical belief systems. Instead I mainly identified as a student asking for support for my research as my final project. I listed some positive and helpful effects where we could show that there is a potential for awareness even in comatose patients and that we could relate to them. At the same time it was obvious but not fully explicit that we would not only have to relate differently to people in altered states of consciousness and within ourselves but also to change a broad range of behavior in the field of medicine and nursing, daily routine and practical and especially ethical procedures. So only the tip of the iceberg was visible but all these implications and consequences were present and having an effect on conversations like this.

In this project I had plenty of opportunities and need to heighten my awareness of power, rank, privileges, authority and roles in a field (for more information see Mindell, A., 1995, and Diamond, J., 2004b).

I was more than ever in contact with and also dependent on the support of professors in the field of medicine and psychology and was also working in a hospital with its complex hierarchical structure. Mindell (1995, p. 28) defines rank as the sum of a person's privileges and extends the concept of rank by not only including social status but also psychological and spiritual rank and the understanding that rank is always contextual. In the beginning I was mainly identified with having low social rank being a student asking for support and permission to do my research about a topic which was not wholly welcomed.

In my curriculum vitae they could have seen that I am also a "Heilpraktiker" (German word for a non-medical or alternative practitioner) which could have easily been associated with long-term conflicts between these camps. There were also moments where I identified with the side in comatose patients which suffers from not being seen as a person and not being equally appreciated in comatose or vegetative states. In a way I was reacting to a culture and its representatives that marginalize these experiences. In order to really see, meet and appreciate the other person and their position, to be able to realize my project, to contribute something and to change this situation by bringing more awareness to these dynamics, I also had to see the other person as a part of myself and part of the culture I have grown up in and I am living in.

In order to no longer fight my own low rank and the other person's high rank but to facilitate these dynamics inside and outside, I had to process my own hurt and become more aware of collective structures contributing to it. On the other side I had to become aware of my own rank such as having the privilege to study these issues and to come up with an exciting idea, my psychological rank gained by my training in Process Work and also my spiritual rank gained by having had important experiences which gave me faith and strength to believe and not give up despite all these challenges.

These inner and outer conflicts challenged me to also become aware and identify with my knowledge, skills and experiences in Coma Work and in general to be more capable of facilitating such situations.

After this negative reply from the university clinic I made contact with two large early rehabilitation units and a special nursing home for people in vegetative states. They declined for various reasons. My first idea was to shift the focus in the direction of working with people in acute delirium but the feedback was not positive even though there is a huge research interest in the medical field. After so many months of trying to get into a clinic to implement my research I was on the way to giving up the topic completely.

Then I received a recommendation to ask the head of the department of the Rheinische Landesklinik in Bonn. Good luck and perseverance in writing large number of emails and making phone calls led to a first meeting. First the head of the department Prof. Biniek delegated this meeting to his assistant medical director but finally he joined it. I was excited and very grateful for their interest and the time they made available and for listening to me as someone without much experience of the daily routine on an intensive unit and talking about these research ideas.

Further big hurdles had to be overcome. The ethics committee of the Medical Association of Düsseldorf informed me that the application needed for this research cost 1500 Euro. After some conversation and filing a very detailed application for a reduction or dispensation the fee was fortunately waived. At the same time I received back all ten copies of the whole application with the response that they were not responsible for me since I was neither a physician nor a student of medicine. I was very desperate in this situation. Finally Prof. Biniek took the responsibility for being the head of this research. So that meant that the ethics committee would oversee the application for the research.

Realization of the research

The neurological intensive care unit of this clinic provided eight places (including ventilation) on the intensive care unit (two two-bed rooms and four single-bed rooms), four places in a stroke unit and a bereavement room. Patients' diagnoses covered amongst others: subarachnoid hemorrhage, stroke, epileptic seizure, Guillain-Barré-Syndrome (GBS-Syndrome), multiple sclerosis and meningitis. The staff consisted of neurologists, nurses, physiotherapists, speech-language therapists, social workers and cleaners. A chaplain came once a week or on request.

I worked on the intensive care unit for eight weeks almost full-time. For the following seven months I came specifically for patients taking part in the study. I started work in the morning joining the meeting of physicians of all three wards of this neurologic clinic discussing diagnostic findings in computed tomographies and magnetic resonance imagings. I participated in daily ward rounds, weekly ward rounds of the head of department and of the assistant medical director and in shift handover periods of the nurses. I was wearing the same blue working clothes as the nurses and most of the physicians. In the morning I was mainly in contact with physicians, while in the afternoon I was more connected with the nursing team and meeting patients personally.

Entering the field

I felt very welcomed and after some time also very integrated in the whole team. I felt very privileged to be included in the medical team as well as in the nursing team without belonging to their profession. It was an exceptional and unusual opportunity to get to know about their point of view and intentions and to learn from them. I realized how important it was to also understand, support and relate to their concerns in order to do my work in cooperation with theirs and to take responsibility for the wellbeing of the patients.

Fully arriving in this environment took some time. The kind of background noises, the technical equipment, the atmosphere and especially the smell brought back old memories which I needed to take care of in myself. Patients not only comatose but also ventilated and analgo-sedated, neuroimaging showing patients' extensive intracerebral mass bleedings and destroyed brain tissues and physicians' matter-of-fact discussions of diagnostic findings, altered my enthusiasm into more and more resignation and hopelessness concerning my research for a while.

I felt like an alien in foreign territory having lost connection to my basis and the world I came from. This paradigm clash created a slight shock in me and I started to lose hope and to doubt if it would be possible at all to apply my work with such critically ill patients and in these surroundings. In that moment I could not imagine myself there standing still next to a patient's bed, meditating, going into altered states of consciousness, loudly framing and appreciating patients' minimal signals or experimenting with movements or even with sounds as something natural and needed in such a situation.

Later I could recognize even more clearly how these processes were not only personal but also a result and expression of our culture and its biomedical model of health and disease where we predominantly marginalize or split off our whole internal worlds and the potential meaningfulness of altered states of consciousness.

A life-threatening situation and especially on an intensive care unit where all vital signs need to be monitored and vital functions are sometimes artificially sustained tends to strongly amplify this polarization and marginalization.

I had underestimated this venture and its collective dimensions. From a system theory point of view I could have been more prepared for the idea that I myself would be the first "comatose patient" to work with and in the next step I would need to put my focus on facilitating the system that I would enter, before I would even met a comatose patient at the bedside. Such preparation could not only have enabled me to more easily facilitate interactions in the system but also to be less caught in unconscious identification with various roles in the field, and as a result experience less suffering and loss of energy. So I had to continue growing on the way.

I needed time to understand and relate to their world, to build up relationships and get familiar with the staff and with the environment. In order to support the research I put up a description of my study on the notice board visible for everybody. I used every opportunity to get in personal contact with nurses and physicians to explain my project, to build up relationships and to identify more with my research. I knew that I would not be able to really do this work while still being completely out of place.

Today I would additionally try to find a space to give a brief introduction in a meeting set up by the head of the department and the head of the nursing service to get more support and to also connect with both professions.

Not belonging to any of these professions gave me some freedom to follow my research interest but also required extra effort to make contact with them. My interest and appreciation for their work and also lending a hand created more and more relationship and support and also great learning for me.

Challenges in the realization of the research

The size of the neurological intensive care unit and the research criteria for the comatose patients led to a very small number of patients available. This was compounded by the unpredictable and sometimes "fast changing" dynamics in the intensive care unit which is just the opposite of what is expected in an empirical study, namely controlled research conditions. I had hoped to have enough access to comatose patients without ventilation and analgo-sedation, in order to have easier access to the patient's awareness within the extremely deep altered state of consciousness, and in consequence to also document minimal signals in a videotape recording.

Since this was not the case I had either give up or also include analgo-sedated patients as has been done in other efficacy studies on coma rehabilitation methods. I decided to include ventilated and analgo-sedated patients, in each case with the physician's agreement, knowing that I could probably not expect strong reactions and having to work against an artificial resistance. That was a challenging and frustrating prospect and in addition a loss of the overt behavior as an outcome variable and a contamination of causal conditions: coma due to medical reason and/or to analgo-sedation.

Various technical problems led to the situation that only the third piece of equipment yielded results which could be evaluated. It was planned to evaluate the heart rate variability and the skin conductivity. However the heart rate revealed too many artifacts to be evaluated probably due in part to limitations in the off-line recording of the measuring instrument and in part due to the critical condition of the patients and their high average age (76.3 years).

Entering and joining altered states of consciousness

Stepping into the role and activity of a researcher moved me even further away from my intention to join patients' experiences at first. I found it an enormous challenge explaining my request to patients' relatives and legal surrogates and getting consent from them, arranging and involving a neurologist conducting a Glasgow Coma Scale assessment, arranging the time for the trial with nurses, assembling the technical equipment consisting of a camcorder on an extra high tripod, a trolley with computer, monitor, physiological-medical instrument, fixing all the electrodes on the patient (three for EEG, two for electrodermal activity), trying to take control of the situation but also to deal with unpredictable disturbances and being aware of the patients' other physiological parameters, as well as staying present and centered and able to join the patients and their experiences.

These conditions activated inner and sometimes also outer expectations exacerbating the feelings of pressure I had to deal with. My understanding and appreciation for the staff's striving for personal contact with patients while constantly having to pay attention to technical equipment and to take care of documentation, grew even more.

There are not many situations in which physiological parameters and processes are so highly controlled and where at the same time the state of consciousness is extremely deep, altered and seemingly out of reach; enormous activity in the surroundings and almost no visible outer activity in the patient and a huge chasm in between.

The transformation required of the researcher in order to transcend this polarization and dualism and enter an extended, heightened and postformal state of consciousness (Wilber, 1997) is a tour de force. This was a further enormous challenge.

I have never felt so strongly thrown back on myself as when I was with someone who was comatose and additionally analgo-sedated. Experiencing little or no contact in such moments made me also aware of my own edges towards altered states, intense feelings and non-doing and my lack of contact to myself. I had to recognize my way of "sedating" myself such as eating too much or keeping myself busy in order to not feel for example. Further personal work, especially on my own past trauma, helped me to get more deeply in contact with myself and to open up to people in comatose or vegetative states.

Again the tendency to be active, to work hard, to be responsible and to have edges to expressing feelings was not just a personal process and due to the momentary situation but also a shared process and dreamt up reaction. When I had the chance to talk in more detail with relatives about the patient's life and attitudes I often heard descriptions such as people being very active, not resting, taking a lot of responsibility for things and showing indications of depression. These psychodynamics are often observed (Mindell, 1999; Reis, 2004) and need further research.

When I managed to become aware of these dynamics and to step out of them I became more detached and present within myself and could more easily invite, accompany and support the patient to follow her processes, without having to do anything or to get anywhere, feeling her feelings or following whatever was important in that moment. In consequence the atmosphere changed, the relationship became more intimate and I also observed that a comatose and analgo-sedated patient would suddenly start to breathe more actively instead of being completely ventilated by the machine.

I was really surprised when I saw patients who had totally given up breathing under ventilation and then during a Process-oriented Coma Work session started to breathe by themselves more actively again, which was also visible on the monitor. Moments like this encouraged me and helped me to develop more faith in the potential for awareness in the deepest states of consciousness.

I was mainly involved with and gained most experience with comatose people without analgo-sedation such as described in appendix I and, outside the clinic, with people in vegetative states. Compared with these, the work with people under analgo-sedation was much more subtle and required more focus on the essence level.

Minimal signals appeared less often. And instead, noticing and trusting changes in the atmosphere and framing them became more important. Introducing myself, framing my intention, having them experience being seen and appreciated as a person going through intense experiences, providing a sense of orientation, encouraging them to believe in all their processes and the importance of them and giving feedback to signals and changes helped to establish a deep rapport.

Apart from at the beginning of the session when I started to talk and approach them by name, I did not refer to their identity by using their name, in order to more easily support entering new experiences. Likewise I had to remind myself not to fall into Process Work jargon when amplifying people's processes but to be aware of my use of language and as far as possible adapt to the person's background.

My attitude towards altered states was even more challenged on a deeper level when I realized at a certain moment that a part of me no longer wanted to enter the intensive care unit to do this work.

I had various reasons for experiencing a resistance and lack of motivation because of facing all these problems such as recurring technical faults, unpredictable changes, lack of support and also an initial conflict with a physician about the sense in working with analgo-sedated patients but I also did not feel fully welcomed with my interest in altered states of consciousness and in comatose patients' experiences. I realized the complexity of the situation.

At first I attributed this reaction to a dislike in the background on the part of the staff towards my project and to experiencing a personal conflict. On another level I thought of this reaction as being a dreamed up reaction in the role of a patient and not being appreciated and welcomed for experiencing altered states of consciousness and not being seen as a person any more, which would mirror a potential conflict between patients and the staff.

A third aspect consisted of further edges towards altered states within myself and a tendency to marginalize my suffering from working hard on gaining measurable results and trying to deal with all these issues.

I think all these and probably other possibilities were true at the same time and apart from my doing inner work on all these roles within myself it would have been a great opportunity to initiate a group process for us all to gain more awareness. I deeply believe if we as caregivers become more aware and gain a deeper connection to our own altered states and their meaningfulness in coma will feel better and recover more easily.

Meeting beyond sedation and at the end of life

Many experiences during this project had a strong impact on me and revealed other aspects and possibilities but were not part of the immediate research. I will mention two of them.

Experiences in working with comatose patients under analgo-sedation mentioned above encouraged me to work with a man in a terminal stage who had already been on the intensive care unit for several weeks. At first I hesitated to work with him because he was on a very high dose of analgo-sedation (Sufenta™ and Dormicum™) partially also due to the fact that people start to adapt to the analgo-sedation after a while. His deeply comatose and strongly sedated state was mirrored in minimal reactions to nursing procedures.

I stood at the bedside and started to meditate. After a while I entered an altered state of consciousness and a state of heightened awareness with a sense of openness and wide and deep contact. I spoke to him and supported him to deeply trust in and follow all his experiences. There developed an atmosphere which I am not able to express in words. It felt as though we were having a profound encounter on another level of reality and as the intensity grew I had a not only goose pimples on my arms, which I sometimes experience, but all over my body. During that short period of time he moved his head very slightly three or four times. I was strongly touched and moved! He died the next day, I hope peacefully.

The other situation happened when I was with an elderly woman who was dying. She was with another patient in a two-bed room in this intensive care unit. A lot of activity was going on at the other bed. In that moment a chaplain came for his weekly visit.

He came also to visit this woman and made contact with her holding her hand, I stood at the foot of the bed. The chaplain and I were communicating by just looking at each other and together we were joining her and holding the space. In the midst of all the action in the room especially due to nurses' and physicians' work at the other bed, I connected to a deep silence and extended state of consciousness full of peacefulness and lightness. It was a blessing and godsend to accompany and witness her dying process.

A path of compassion

When I reviewed my impulse to work with people in comatose states on an intensive care unit instead of working with people in vegetative states in special nursing homes for the project, I had another realization.

I remembered that the reasons why I chose the first situation were that I thought it would be easier because I would be able to use the equipment already there such as the ECG monitor and I would have the support of neurologists conducting a Glasgow Coma Scale assessment.

Despite these understandable reasons I realized deeper motivations that I had marginalized. I noticed an ambitious tendency to want to demonstrate something remarkable which probably was less likely with people in vegetative states. People in vegetative states might not show huge reactions or even might never wake up. Today I know that it is absolutely not true and that working with people under analgo-sedation can be more challenging than working with people in vegetative or minimal states of consciousness. But more important and shocking was the inherent marginalization and dismissiveness in my attitude towards people in vegetative states and towards a part in myself that expresses a system of values which only appreciates people when they are productive and achieving something instead of loving people simply for their presence as a human being.

I was deeply affected and cried for quite a while about the suffering and pain such an attitude has been creating and supporting in people and in myself. This experience fundamentally changed my attitude not only towards people in vegetative states but also towards those with disabilities. I started to open up more to people's suffering in the past and present and to allow more intense feelings to arise. In time I realized how it helped me to also become more compassionate with myself.

Reaching out to people in comatose states led to a path of compassion. In order to make contact with people who seemed to be lost in unknown states I had to explore more deeply my own unknown and altered states of consciousness and edges to enter them.

I noticed more often moments where I was totally absorbed in following ambitious tendencies in order to overcome internal lack of self-worth which in consequence led to feelings of isolation, a sense of being stuck and hopelessness.

My goal of completing my studies in psychology and Process Work sometimes aggravated this dynamic but in the long run helped to become more aware and to step out of this pattern. My work with people in comatose states played a large role in this development. Meeting them in extremely deep altered states of consciousness, appreciating them just for their presence as loving human beings and trusting their minimal signals as an expression of awareness helped me to meet and relate to them, to the world and to myself more deeply.

"If you want others to be happy, practice compassion. If you want to be happy, practice compassion."

14th Dalai Lama, Tenzin Gyatso

"Through the Thou a person becomes I."

Martin Buber

ABSTRACT

This research is an extensive survey and the first explorative empirical study of awareness in comatose states and the possibility of contact and communication with comatose patients in a neurological intensive care unit setting using Process-oriented Coma Work methods developed by Arnold Mindell.

The study provides present-day definitions and comparisons of terms such as coma, vegetative state, minimally conscious state, locked-in syndrome and psychogenic unresponsiveness in the field of neuroscience. Standard definitions of consciousness and its assessment by coma scales, coma scoring systems and neurological correlates are be presented. Findings of comatose and vegetative state patients' ability not only to hear (sensation) but also to understand meaning (perception) are presented. A survey of studies on patients' reports after a period of unconsciousness shows evidence for awareness in so-called unconscious states. Studies which have surveyed diagnostic accuracy in respect of vegetative state and minimally conscious state in recent years show up to 43% of misdiagnosis and reveal the challenge of assessing disorders of consciousness. A survey of most relevant recent findings of evidence of consciousness in coma, vegetative state and minimally conscious state and also reports on late improvement from vegetative state and minimally conscious state are reported. A further investigation of consciousness revisiting the definitions, basic assumptions and current basic questions are shared. Wilber's integral theory of consciousness, Tart's concept of altered states of consciousness and Mindell's dreambody and field concepts are explained to come to a deeper understanding and wider concept of consciousness and to the Process-oriented approach to people in comatose states. A short overview of rehabilitation methods is followed by a description of Process-oriented Coma Work and its basic assumptions, methods and application. All strands presented lead to an integral Process-oriented approach to people in comatose states: different approaches to consciousness are set in a wider context, philosophical, cultural and ethical aspects and their consequences are discussed and finally the Process-oriented approach to comatose people is explored from a personal, relationship, environmental and field point of view.

Effects of Process-oriented Coma Work interventions and Arnold Mindell's assumptions on which they are based were tested. Mindell assumes that coma is not a state of absence of consciousness as defined in neuroscience but an extremely deep altered state of consciousness in which there is potential for awareness. Contact and communication can be established by radically related Process-oriented Coma Work interventions.

It was assumed that Process-oriented interventions will lead to an increase in skin conductance level and skin conductance responses compared to a baseline measurement and that these interventions will lead to a higher increase than during the coma depth assessment. Coma depth was assessed by the Glasgow Coma Scale (score of <8). From the 16 patients who took part in the research 7 were included in the study.

The results confirm the four hypotheses: 1. Skin conductance level (SCL) significantly increased in the intervention compared to the baseline. 2. The increase in SCL during Process-oriented Coma Work intervention was greater than during Glasgow Coma Scale assessment. 3. Skin conductance responses (SCR) showed highly significant results during Process-oriented intervention compared to the baseline. 4. The increase in SCR during Process-oriented Coma Work intervention was greater than during Glasgow Coma Scale assessment.

This dynamic mirrors an increase of chronological integration of processes in different compartments of neuronal activity which is a neurological correlate, a presupposition of consciousness and a precursor of overt behavior. The results show evidence for awareness in comatose patients and for Process-oriented coma interventions as a valid coma rehabilitation method.

Finally limitations, strengths, implications and recommendations for further research are discussed.

Appendix I comprises a translated verbatim transcription of a Process-oriented Coma Work session with a non-sedated but comatose patient (Glasgow Coma Score: 4 points) which could not be included in the evaluation of the study. The transcript documents the patient's behavior during the baseline phase, the interaction in the Glasgow Coma Scale assessment phase and the interaction and the awakening of the patient during the Process-oriented Coma Work intervention phase.

Appendix II presents a counterpart and complement to the empirical research including reflections, personal experiences, processes and developments during the preparation and realization of this project.

LIST OF ABBREVIATIONS

Abbreviation:	Definition:
ABR	Auditory brain-stem response
ASC	Altered state of consciousness
CR	Consensus reality
CRS-R	Coma Recovery Scale Revised
CT	Computed tomography
EDA	Electrodermal activity
EEG	Electroencephalogram
ERP	event-related brain potential
GCS	Glasgow Coma Scale
GOS	Glasgow Outcome Scale
LIS	Locked-In syndrome
MCS	Minimally conscious state
MEG	Magnetoencephalographic
MR Mini	mal responsive patient
MRI, fMRI	(functional) Magnetic resonance imaging
NCR	Nonconsensus reality
PET	Positron emission tomography
PVS	Persistent vegetative state
SCL	Skin conductance level
SCR	Skin conductance response
VS	Vegetative state

REFERENCES

Aldrige, D., Gustorff, D. & Hannich, H. J. (1990). Where am I? Music therapy applied to coma patients. *Journal of the Royal Society of Medicine,* 83: 345-346

Amercian Academy of Neurology (1989). Position of the AAN on certain aspects of the care and management of the persistent vegetative state patient: adopted by the executive board. American Academy of *Neurology,* April 21, 1988, Cincinnati, Ohio. Neurology, 39: 125-126

American Congress of Rehabilitation Medicine (1995). Recommendations for use of uniform nomenclature pertinent to patients with sever alterations in consciousness. *Archives of Physical Medicine and Rehabilitation,* 76: 205-209

Andrews, K. (1993). Recovery of patients after four months or more in the persistent vegetative state. *British Medical Journal,* 306: 1597-1600

Andrews, K. (1996). International working party on the management of the vegetative state. *Brain Injury,* 10 (11): 797-806

Andrews, K., Murphy, L., Munday, R. & Littlewood, C. (1996). Misdiagnosis of the vegetative state: retrospective study in a rehabilitation unit. *British Medical Journal,* 313: 13-16

Andrews, K. (2004). Medical decision making in the vegetative state: withdrawal of nutrition and hydration. *Neuro Rehabilitation,* 19 (4): 299-304

Arts, W. F. M., van Dongen, H. R., van Hof-van Duin, J., Lammens, E. (1985). Unexpected improvement after prolonged posttraumatic vegetative state. *Journal of Neurology, Neurosurgery & Psychiatry,* 48: 1300-1303

Avanzini, G. (1999). The concept of consciousness: a challenge for the neuroscientist. *Italian Journal of Neurological Science*, 20: 5-6

Bausewein, C., Roller, S. & Voltz, R. (Eds.) (2007). *Leitfaden Palliativmedizin – Palliative Care* (3. ed.). München: Elsevier

Bergblom-Engberg, L., Hallenberg, B., Wickstrom, I. & Haljamae, H. (1988). A retrospective study of patients recall of respirator treatment. *Intensive Care Nursing*, 6: 150-160

Block, N. (1995). On a confusion about the function of consciousness. Behavioral and Brain Sciences 18: 227-47. In Güven Güzeldere (1995): Problems of consciousness: a perspective on contemporary issues, current debates. *Journal of consciousness studies*, 2 (1): 112-143

Boly, M., Faymonville, M. E., Peigneux, P., Lambermont, B., Damas, P., Del Fiore, G., Degueldre, C., Franck, G., Luxen, A., Lamy, M., Moonen, G., Maquet, P., Laureys, S. (2004). Auditory processing in severely brain injuried patients: differences between the minimally consciousness state and the persistent vegetative state. *Archives of Neurology*, 61: 233-238

Bortz, J. (1993). *Statistik für Sozialwissenschaftler* (4th ed.). Berlin: Springer

Bortz, J., Lienert, G. A. & Boehnke, K. (2008). *Verteilungsfreie Methoden in der Biostatistik*. Berlin: Springer

Boucsein, W. (1988). *Elektrodermale Aktivität*. Berlin: Springer

Bozza Marrubini, M. (1984). Classifications of coma. *Intensive Care Medicine*, 10: 217-26

Cartlidge, N. (2001). States related to or confused with coma. *Journal of Neurology, Neurosurgery & Psychiatry*, 71 (suppl. I): i18-i19

Celesia, G. G. (1993). Persistent vegetative state: report of the American Neurological Association Committee on ethical affairs. *Annals of Neurology*, 33 (4): 386–390

Chalmers, D. (1995). The puzzle of consciousness experience. *Scientific American*, 237 (6): 62-68

Childs, N. L., Mercer, W. N. & Childs, H. W. (1993). Accuracy of diagnosis of persistent vegetative state. *Neurology*, 43: 1465-67

Childs, N. L. & Mercer, W. N. (1996). Late improvement in consciousness after post-traumatic vegetative state. *New England Journal of Medicine*, 334, 24-25

Chögyal Namkhai Norbu (2002). *Dream yoga and the practice of natural light*. Boulder, CO: Snow Lion Publications

Collopy, M. (2002). *Architects of peace: visions of hope in words and images*. Novato, CA.: New World Library

Dennett, D. (1987). Consciousness. In R. L. Gregory (ed.), *The Oxford Companion to the Mind* (pp. 160-164). Oxford: Oxford University Press

Di, H. B., Yu, S. M., Weng, X. C., Laureys, S., Yu, D., Li, J. Q., Qin, P. M., Zhu, Y. H., Zhang, S. Z. & Chen, Y. Z. (2007). Cerebral response to patient's own name in the vegetative and minimally conscious state. *Neurology*, 68: 895-899

Diamond, J. & Jones, L. S. (2004a). *A path made by walking: process work in practice*. Portland, OR.: Lao Tse Press

Diamond, J. (2004b). Where roles, rank and relationship meet: a framework for working with multiple role relationships in process work learning communities. Unpublished article, retrieved December, 14, 2008, from: http://www.juliediamond.net/resources.php

Ekman, P. & Friesen, W. V. (1976). *Facial Action Coding System: A Technique for the Measurement of Facial Movement*. Palo Alto, CA.: Consulting Psychologists Press

Fischer, C., Morlet, D., Bouchet, P., Luaute, J., Jourdan, C. & Salord, F. (1999). Mismatch negativity and late auditory evoked potentials in comatose patients. *Clinical Neurophysiology*, 110: 1601-1610

Freemon, F. R. (1971). Akinetic mutism and bilateral anterior cerebral occlusion. *Journal of Neurology, Neurosurgery & Psychiatry*, 34: 693-698

Gerstenbrand, F. (1967). *Das Traumatische apallische Syndrom: Klinik, Morphologie, Pathophysiologie und Behandlung*. Springer: Wien

Giacino, J. T. & Zasler, N. D. (1995). Outcome after severs traumatic brain injury: coma, the vegetative state, and the minimally responsive state. *Journal of Head Trauma Rehabilitation*, 10, 1: 40-56

Giacino, J. T., Zasler, N. D., Katz, D. I., Kelly, J. P., Rosenberg, J. H. & Filley, C. M. (1997). Development of practice guidelines for assessment and management of the vegetative and minimal conscious states. *Journal of Head Trauma Rehabilitation*, 12 (4): 79-89

Giacino, J. T., Ashwal, S., Childs, N., Cranford, R., Jennet, B., Katz, D. I., Kelly, J. P., Rosenberg, J. H., Whyte, J., Zafonte, R. D. & Zasler, N. D. (2002). The minimal conscious state: definition and diagnostic criteria. *American Academy of Neurology*, 58: 349-353

Giacino, J. T. (2004). The vegetative and minimally conscious states: consensus-based criteria for establisihing diagnosis and prognosis. *Neuro Rehabilitation*, 19: 293-298

Gott, P. S., Rabinovicz, A. L., DiGiorgio, C. M. (1991). P300 auditory event-related potentials in nontraumatic coma: association with Glasgow Coma Scale and awakening. *Archives of Neurology*, 48: 1267-1270

Gramann, K. & Schandry, R. (2009). *Psychophysiologie. Körperliche Indikatoren psychischen Geschehens.* (4th revised edition). Weinheim: Beltz

Guerit, J. M., Verougstraete, D., Tourtchaninoff, M., Debatisse, D., Witdoeckt, C. (1999). ERPs obtained with the auditory oddball paradigm in coma and altered states of consciousness: clinical relationships prognostic value and origin of components. *Clinical Neurophysiology*, 110: 1260-1269

Gustorf, D. & Hannich, H.-J. (1992). *Jenseits des Wortes: Musiktherapie mit komatösen Patienten auf der Intensivstation.* Bern: Huber

Güzeldere, G. (1995a). Consciousness: what it is, how to study it, what to learn from its history. *Journal of consciousness studies*, 2,1: 30-51

Güzeldere, G. (1995b). Problems of consciousness: a perspective on contemporary issues, current debates. *Journal of consciousness studies*, 2 (1): 112-143

Habermas, J. (1979). Communication and the evolution of society. Trans. and intro. Thomas McCarthy. Boston: Beacon. In Ken Wilber (1997): an integral theory of consciousness. *Journal of Consciousness Studies*, 4 (1), 71-92

Hagen, C., Malkmus, D. & Durham, P. (1979). *Levels of cognitive functioning. Rehabilitation of the head injuried adult: comprehensive physical management.* Dowey, CA: Professional Staff Association of the Rancho Los Amigos Hospital, Inc.

Hamel, M. B., Goldman, L., Teno, J., Lynn, J., Davis, R. B., Harrell, F. E., Connors, A. F., Califf, R., Kussin, P.; Bellamy, P. et al. (1995). Identification of comatose patients at high risk for death or severe disability. Support investigators. Understand prognoses and preferences for outcomes and risks of treatments. *Journal of American Medical Association*, 273 (23): 1842-8

Hannich, H.-J. (2009). Psychosomatische Aspekte der Intensivmedizin. In Thure von Uexküll & Rolf Adler (eds.), *Psychosomatische Medizin: Modelle ärztlichen Denkens und Handelns* (unpublished pre-printed version). München: Urban & Fischer

Heindl, U. T. & Laub, M. C. (1996). Outcome of persistent vegetative state following hypoxic or traumatic brain injury in children and adolescents. *Neuropediatrics*, 27: 94-100

Herkenrath, A. (2006). Musiktherapie in der Langzeitphase des Wachkomas – Aspekte zur Evaluation von Wahrnehmung und Bewusstsein. *Neurologie & Rehabilitation*, 12, 1: 22-32

Higashi, K., Hatano, M., Abiko, S., Ihara, K., Katayama, S., Wakuta, Y., Okamura, T. & Yamashita, T. (1981). Five-year follow-up study of patients with persistent vegetative state. *Journal of Neurology, Neruosurgery & Psychiatry*, 44 (6): 552-554

Hildebrandt, H., Zieger, A., Engel, A. , Fritz, K. W. & Bussmann,

B. (1998). Differentiation of autonomic nervous activity in different stages of coma displayed by power spectrum analysis of heart rate variability. *European Archives of Psychiatry & Clinical Neuroscience*, 248: 46-52

Hildebrandt, H., Zieger, A., Engel, A. & Kraft, A. (1999). Kardiosomatische Kopplung als differentieller Indikator für Komatiefe und Effektivität sensorischer Stimulation. *Aktuelle Neurologie*, 26: 171-179

Hinder, F., Skopp, G. & Van Aken, H. (2001). Koma. In: H. van Aken, K. Reinhart & M. Zimpfer (Eds.), *Intensivmedizin* (pp. 962-991). Stuttgart: Thieme

Jennet, B. & Plum, F. (1972). Persistent vegetative state after brain damage: a syndrome looking for a name. *Lancet*, 1: 734-737

Jennet, B. (2002). *The vegetative state: medical facts, ethical and legal dilemma*. Cambridge: Cambridge University Press

Jung, C. G. (1991). *Praxis der Psychotherapie. Praxis der Psychotherapie: Beiträge zum Problem der Psychotherapie und zur Psychologie der Übertragung* (Vol. XVI). Olten: Walter

Kane, N. M., Butler, S. R. & Simpson, T. (2000). Coma outcome prediction using event-related potentials: P3 and mismatching negativity. *Audiology and Neuro-Otology*, 5: 186-191

Kassubek, J., Juengling, F. D., Els, T. et al. (2003). Activation of a residual cortical network during painful stimulation in long-term postanoxic vegetative state: a 150-H20 PET study. *Journal of Neurological Science*, 212: 85-91

Kolb, B. & Wishaw, I. Q. (2003). *Human Neuropsycholoy* (5th editon). New York: Worth Publishers

Kotchoubey, B., Lang, S., Bostanov, V. & Birnbaumer, N. (2002). Is there a mind? Electrophysiology of unconscious patients. *News in Physiological Science*, 17: 38-42

Kretschmer, E. (1940). Das apallische Syndrom. Zeitschrift für die gesamte *Neurologie und Psychiatrie*, 169: 576-579

LaBerge, S. (1990). Psychophysiological studies of consciousness during sleep. In R.R. Bootzen, J.F. Kihlstrom &

D.L. Schacter (eds.), *Sleep and Cognition* (pp. 109-126). Washington, DC: American Psychological Association

Lancaster, B. L. (1997). On stages of perception: towards a synthesis of cognitive neuroscience and the Buddhist abhidhamma tradition. *Journal of Consciousness*, 4 (2): 122-42

Lanzerath, D. (1998). Koma, irreversibles/irreversible Komatöse, „2. ethisch". In W. Korff, L. Beck, P. Mikat (eds.), *Lexikon der Bioethik* (Vol. 2, 410-412). Gütersloh: Görres-Gesellschaft

La Puma, J., Schiedermayer, D. L., Gulyas, A. E. & Siegler, M. (1988). Talking to comatose patients. *Archives of Neurology.*, Jan.; 45 (1): 20-22

Laureys, S., Boly, M., Maquet, P. (2006). Tracking the recovery of consciousness from coma. *Journal Clinical Investigation*, 116: 1823-1825

Laureys, S., Faymonville, M. E., Deguledre, C., Del Fiore, G., Damas, P., Lambermonr, B., Janssens, N., Aerts, J., Franck, G., Luxen, A., Moonen, G., Lamy, M. & Maquet, P. (2000a). Auditory processing in the vegetative state. *Brain*, 123: 1589-1601

Laureys, S., Faymonville, M. E., Luxen, A., Lamy, M., Franck, G., Maquet, P. (2000b). Restoration of thalamocortical connectivity after recovery from persistent vegetative state. *Lancet*, 355: 1790-1791

Laureys, S., Faymonville, M. E., Peigneux, P., Damas, P., Lambermont, B., Del Fiore, G., Degueldre, C., Aerts, J., Luxen, A., Franck, G., Lamy, M., Moonen, G., Maquet, P. (2002). Cortical processing of noxious somatosensory stimuli in the persistent vegetative state. *Neuroimage*, 17: 732-741

Laureys, S., Faymonville, M. E., De Tiège, X., Peigneux, P., Berré, J., Moonen, G., Goldman, S., Maquet, P. (2004). Brain function in the vegetative state. *Advances in Experimental Medicine and Biology*, 550: 229-38

Laureys, S. (2006). Tracking the recovery of consciousness from coma. *Journal of Clinical Investigation*, 116: 1823-1825

Laureys, S., Boly, M. (2007). What is it like to be vegetative or minimally conscious? *Neurology*, 20: 609-13

Laureys, S. (2008). Wach und doch bewusstlos. Mit raffinierten Gehirnaufnahmen können Neurologen heute das Wachkoma und seine Übergangsformen zuverlässiger diagnostizieren. *Spektrum der Wissenschaft*, 3: 44-49

Lawrence, M. (1995). The unconscious experience. *American Journal of Critical Care*, 3: 227-232

Leuwer, M., Trappe, H..J., Schürmeyer, T. H. & Zuzan, O. (2004). *Checkliste Interdisziplinäre Intensivmedizin* (2nd edition). Stuttgart: Thieme

Levy, D. E., Bates, D., Caronna, J. J., Cartlidge, N. E., Knill-Jones, R. P., Lapinski, R. H., Singer, B. H., Shaw, D. A. & Plum, F. (1981). Prognosis in nontraumatic coma. *Annals of Internal Medicine*, 94: 293-301.

Ludwig, A. M. (1969). Altered states of consciousness. In Charles Tart (ed.), *Altered states of consciousness: a book of readings* (p. 9-22). New York: Wiley.

Ludwig, Christian A. (2000). Flüssigkeitssubstitution in der Terminalphase. In Eberhard Aulbert & Detlev Zech (Eds.), *Lehrbuch der Palliativmedizin*. Stuttgart: Schattauer

Matsuda, W., Matsumura, A., Komatsu, Y., Yanaka, K. & Nose, T. (2003). Awakenings from persisent vegetative state: report of three cases with parkinson and brain stem lesions on MRI. *Journal of Neurology, Neurosurgery & Psychiatry*, 74: 1571-1573

Mindell, Amy (1995). *Metaskills: the spiritual art of therapy*. Las Vegas, NV: New Falcon Publications

Mindell, Amy (1999). *Coma – a healing journey: a guide for family, friends and helpers*. Portland, Oregon: Lao Tse Press

Mindell, Arnold (1985). *The Dreambody: Körpersymbole als Sprache der Seele*. Fellbach-Oeffingen: Bonz

Mindell, Arnold (1985). *River's way: process science of the dream body*. London: Routledge & Kegan Paul

Mindell, Arnold (1987). *The dreambody in relationships.* New York: Penguin

Mindell, Arnold (1989). *Coma: key to awaking. working with the dreambody near death.* New York, Penguin-Arkana

Mindell, Arnold (1992). *The leader as martial artist: techniques and strategies for resolving conflict and creating community.* San Francisco: Harper Collins

Mindell, Arnold (1995). *Sitting in the fire: large group transformation through diversity and conflict.* Portland, OR.: Lao Tse Press

Mindell Arnold (2000). *Quantum mind: the edge between physics and psychology.* Portland, OR.: Lao Tse Press

Mindell, Arnold (2004). *The quantum mind and Healing: how to listen and respond to your body's symptoms.* Charlottesville, VA: Hampton

Monti, M., Vanhaudenhuyse, A., Coleman, M. R., Boly, M., Pickard, J. D., Tshibanda, L., Owen, A. M. & Laureys S. (2010). Willful modulation of brain activity in disorders of consciousness. *New England Journal of Medicine,* 362: 579-589

Multi-Society Task Force on PVS (1994). Medical aspects of PVS: statement of the Multi-Society Task Force. Part I. *New England Journal of Medicine,* 330 (21): 1499-1508

Multi-Society Task Force on PVS (1994). Medical aspects of PVS: statement of the Multi-Society Task Force. Part II. *New England Journal of Medicine,* 330 (21), 1572-1579

Mutschler, V., Chaumeil, C. G., Marcoux, L., Wioland, N., Tempe, J. & Kurtz, D. (1996). Etude du P300 auditif chez des sujets en coma post-anoxique. *Clinical Neurophysiology,* 26: 158-163

Naqvi, N. H., & Bechara, A. (2006). Skin conductance: a psycho¬physiological approach to the study of decision making. In C. Senior, T. Russell & M. S. Gazzaniga (Eds.), *Methods in mind.* The MIT Press

Niedermeyer, E. (1999). A concept of consciousness. I*talian Journal of Neurological Science,* 20, (1): 7-15

Nijenhuis, H. & de Vetten, L. (2006). Coma and Coma Care in South Africa (unpublished study)

Osterbrink, J. H., Mayer, H., Ewers, A., Fiedler, Ch., Haslbeck, J., Wirth, K., Wordel, A., Hannich, H. J., Krian, A., Laczkivics, A., Weyand, M., McDonough, J., Evers, G. (2004). Akute postoperative Verwirrtheit kardiochirurgischer Patienten. *Zeitschrift für ärztliche Fortbildung und Qualität im Gesundheitswesen*, 98 (9): 761-765

Owen, A. M., Coleman, M. R., Davis, M. H., Boly, M., Laureys, S., Pickard, J. D. (2006). Detecting awareness in the vegetative state. *Science*, 313 (5792): 1402

Owen, A. M., Coleman, M. R., Davis, M. H., Boly, M., Laureys, S. & Pickard, J. D. (2007): Using functional magnetic resonance imaging to detect covert awareness in the vegetative state. *Archives of Neurology*, 64, 1098-1102

Plum, F. & Posner, J. B. (1966). *The diagnosis of stupor and coma*. Philadelphia: FA Davis

Plum, F. & Posner, J. B. (1982). *The diagnosis of stupor and coma* (3rd ed). Philadelphia: FA Davis

Podurgiel, M. (1990). The unconscious experience – a pilot study. Journal of *Neuroscience Nursing*, 22 (1): 52-53

Posner, J. B., Saper, C. B., Schiff, N. D. & Plum, F. (2007). P*lum and Posner's diagnosis of stupor and coma*. Oxford: University Press

Prasad, K. (1996). The Glasgow Coma Scale: a critical appraisal of its clinimetric properties. *Journal of Clinical Epidemiology*, 49(7): 755-63

Rappport, M., Hall, K. M. et al. (1982). Disability rating scale for severe head trauma: coma to community. *Archives Physical Medicine and Rehabilitation*, 63: 118-123

Reiss, G. (2004). *Vital loving: a guide book for couples and families*. Eugene, OR.: Changing Worlds Publications

Reuter, B. M., Linke, D. D., Kurthen, M. (1989). Kognitive Prozesse bei Bewusstlosen? Eine Brain-Mapping-Studie zu P 300. *Archives of Psychology*, 141: 155-173

Rosenberg, G. A., Johnson, S. F. & Brenner, R. P. (1977). Recovery of cognition after prolonged vegetative state. *Annals of*

Neurology, 2: 167-168

Rosenblath, W. (1899). Über einen bemerkenswerten Fall von Hirnerschütterung (aus dem Landeskrankenhaus Kassel). *Archiv für Klinische Medizin*, 64: 406-424

Royal College of Physicians of London (2003). The vegetative state. Guidance on diagnosis and management.

Rundshagen, K. Schnabel, C. Wegner & Schulte, J. am Esch (2002). Incidence of recall, nightmares, and hallucinations during analgo-sedation in intensive care. *Intensive Care Medicine*; 28 (1): 38-43

Russell, S. (1999). An exploratory study of patient's perceptions, memories and experiences of an intensive care unit. *Journal of Advanced Nursing*, 29: 783-791

Sakamoto, Hitomi (2004). Caregivers' experience of Process-oriented Coma Work: a phenomenological study. (Doctoral) Dissertation Abstracts International, 66-03B. Retrieved Dezember, 20, 2009, from: http://gateway.proquest. com/openurl?url_ver=Z39.88-2004&rft_val_fmt=info: ofi/fmt:kev:mtx:dissertation&res_dat=xri:pqdiss&rft_ dat=xri:pqdiss:3168558

Scharfetter, C. (1996). *Allgemeine Psychopathologie: Eine Einführung* (4th ed.). Stuttgart: Thieme

Schelling, G.., Stoll, C., Haller, M., Briegel, J., Manert, W., Hummel, T., Lenhart, A., Heyduck, M., Polasek, J., Meier, W., Peter, K. (1998). Health-related quality of life and posttraumatic stress disorder in survivors of the acute respiratory distress syndrome. *Critical Care Medicine*, 26: 651-659

Schelling, G., Peter, K. (2006). Stress, emotionales Gedächtnis und gesundheitsbezogene Lebensqualität bei Patienten nach Intensivtherapie. In Thomas Kammerer (Ed.), *Traumland Intensivstation – Veränderte Bewusstseinszustände und Koma. Interdisziplinäre Expeditionen*. Norderstedt: Books on Demand

Schiff, N. D., Ribary, U., Moreno, D. R., Beattie, B., Kronberg, E.,

Blasberg, R., Giacino, J., McCagg, C., Fins, J., Llinás, R. & Plum, F. (2002). Residual cerebral activity and behavioral fragments can remain in the persistent vegetative brain. *Brain*, 125: 1210-1234

Schiff, N. D., Rodriguez-Moreno, D., Kamal, A., Kim, K. H. S., Giacino, J.T., Plum, F. and Hirsch, J. (2005). fMRI reveals large-scale network activation in minimally conscious patients. *Neurology*, 64: 514-523

Schnakers, C., Vanhaudenhuyse, A., Giacino, J., Ventura, M. Boly, M., Majerus, S. Moonen, G. & Laureys, S. (2009). Diagnositc accuracy of the vegetative and minimally conscious state: clinical consensus versus standardized neurobehavioral assessment. *BMC Neurology*, 9:35. DOI: 10.1186/1471-2377-9-35. Retrieved February, 10, 2009, from http://www.biomedcentral.com/1471-2377/9/35

Schnaper, N. (1975). The psychological implications of severe trauma: emotional sequelae to unconsciousness. *Journal of Trauma*, 15 (2): 94-98

Sogyal Rinpoche (1993). *Das tibetische Buch vom Leben und vom Sterben: ein Schlüssel zum tieferen Verständnis von Leben und Tod*. Bern: Barth

Spittler, J. F., Langenstein, P. & Calabrese, P. (1993). Die Quantifizierung krankhafter Bewusstseinsstörungen. Gütekriterien, Zwecke, Handlichkeit. *Anästhesie, Intensivmedizin, Notfallmedizin, Schmerztherapie*, 4, (28): 213-221

Stalhammar, D. & Starmark, J. E. (1986). Assessment of responsiveness in head injury patients. The Glasgow Coma Scale and some comments on alternative methods. *Acta Neurochirurgica*, 36, suppl.: 91-94

Stanczak, D. E., White, J. G., Gouview, W. D., Moehle, K. A., Daniel, M., Novack, T., Long, C. J. (1984). Assessment of responsiveness in acute cerebral disorders. a multicentre study on the reaction level scale (RLS 85). *Acta Neurochirugica*, 90: 73-80

Steuck, J. (1978). Good morning, Judy. Minneapolis: Augsburg Publishing House. In John La Puma, David L. Schiedermayer, Ann E. Gulyas & Mark Siegler (1988). Talking to comatose patients. *Archives of Neurology*, Jan., 45 (1): 20-22

Szirtes, J., Diekmann, V., Kuhwald, H., Hülser, P. J., Jürgens, R. (1990). EEG spectra and evoked potentials to words in apallic patients. In L. Deecke, J. C. Eccles & V. B. Mountcastle (Eds.), *From neuron to action. An appraisal of fundamental and clinical research* (pp. 651-653). Berlin: Springer

Tart, C. (Ed.) (1969). *Altered states of consciousness: a book of readings.* New York: Wiley.

Tart, C. (1972). States of consciousness and state-specific sciences. *Science*, 176: 1203-1210

Tart, C. (1978). *Transpersonale Psychologie.* Olten: Walter.

Tart, C. (1983). *States of consciousness.* New York: Dutton.

Teasdale, G. & Jennett, B. (1974). Assessment of coma and impaired consciousness: a practical scale. *Lancet* 2: 81-84

Tellkamp, A. (2006). Das ideale Intensivzimmer. In T. Kammerer (Ed.), *Traumland Intensivstation: veränderte Bewusstseinszustände und Koma. Interdisziplinäre Expeditionen* (pp. 359-376). Norderstedt: Books on Demand

Thacker, A. K., Singh, B. N., Sarkari, N. B. & Mishra, R. K. (1997). Non-traumatic coma – profile and prognosis. *Journal of Association of Physicians of India*, Apr. 45 (4): 267-70

Todorow, S. (1975). Recovery of children after severe head injury. Psychoreactive superimpositions. *Scandinavian Journal of Rehabilitation Medicine*, 7: 93-96

Todorow. S. (1978). Posttraumatischer pseudokomatöser Zustand: Dornröschen-Stupor bei Kindern. *Hefte Unfallheilkunde*, 132: 245-246

Tosch, P. (1988). Patients recollections of their posttraumatic coma. *Journal of Neuroscience Nursing*, 20: 223-228.

Tranel, D., & Damasio, H. (1994). Neuroanatomical correlates of electrodermal skin-conductance responses. *Psychophysiology*, 31, 427-438

Tresch, D. D., Farrol, H. S., Duthie, E. H., Goldstein, M. D., Lane, P. S. (1991). Clinical characteristics of patients in the persistent vegetative state. *Archives of Internal Medicine*, 151: 900-932

Turner, J. S., Briggs, S. J., Springhorn, H. E., Potgieter, P. D. (1990). Patient's recollection of intensive care unit experience. *Critical Care Medicine*, 18: 966-968

Van der Mast, R. C. (1999). Postoperative delirium. *Dementia and Geriatric Cognitive Disorders*, 10: 401-405

Van Gulick, R. (2009). Consciousness. In *The Stanford Encyclopedia of Philosophy* (Winter 2009 Edition), Edward N. Zalta (ed.), URL = <http://plato.stanford.edu/archives/win2009/entries/consciousness/>

Varela, F. J. (2006). *Traum, Schlaf und Tod. Der Dalai Lama im Gespräch mit westlichen Wissenschaftlern* (5th ed.). München: Piper

Velmans, M. (2002). How could conscious experiences affect brains? *Journal of Consciousness Studies*, 9: 3-29

Voss, H. U., Uluç, A. M., Dyke, J. P., Watts, R., Kobylarz, E. J., McCandliss, B. D., Heier, L. A., Beattie, B. J., Hamacher, K. A., Vallabhajosula, S., Goldsmith, S. J., Ballon, D., Giacino, J.T. & Schiff, N. D. (2006). Possible axonal regrowth in late recovery from the minimally conscious state. *Journal of Clinical Investigation*, 116: 2005-2011

Vossel, G. & Zimmer, H. (1998). *Psychophysiologie* (Vol. 4). Stuttgart: Kohlhammer

Watzlawick, P., Beavin, J. H. & Jackson, D. D. (1996). *Menschliche Kommuni-kation: Formen, Störungen, Paradoxien* (9th ed.). Bern: Huber

Weyermann R (2006). Subjektives Erleben von Körpersymptomen: proessorientierte Entfaltung, Perspektiven und Bedeutungen. Unpublished dissertation, Uni. Basel. Retrieved December, 14, 2009, from:

http://pages.unibas.ch/diss/2006/DissB_7528.htm

Wijdicks, E. F., Bamlet, W. R., Maramattom, B. V., Manno, E. M., McClelland, R. L. (2005). Validation of a new coma scale: the FOUR score. *Annals of Neurology* 58 (4): 585–93

Wilber, K. (1997). An integral theory of consciousness. *Journal of Consciousness Studies*, 4 (1): 71-92

Wilber, K. (2001). *Integrale Psychologie. Geist, Bewusstsein, Psychologie und Therapie.* Freiamt: Arbor

Yagi, T. & Baba, S. (1983). Evaluation of the brainstem functions by the response and the caloric vestibular reaction in the comatose. *Archives of Otorhinolaryngology*, 238 (1): 33-34

Zasler, N. D. (2004). Terminology in evolution: caveats, conundrums and controversies. *NeuroRehabilitation*, 19: 285–292

Zieger, A. & Hildebrandt, H. (1996): Interventionsbegleitende Messungen ereigniskorrelierter autonomer Potentiale während "Koma-Stimulation" nach schwerem Schädel-Hirntrauma: Ein neues Verfahren für Qualitätsmanagement und Evaluation in der Frührehabilitation? In Hedon-Klinik (eds.), *Qualitätsmanagement - neurologische Frührehabilitation. Tagungsband zum 2. Reha-Symposium Neurologie und Orthopädie - Lingener Tage 1996* (pp. 209-231). Münster: Rhema-Verlag

Zieger, A. (1999). Klinische Neurorehabilitation und Neuroethik (unpublished cumulative postdoctoral thesis). Carl von Ossietzky Universität Oldenburg

INDEX

A

ABOUT THE AUTHOR

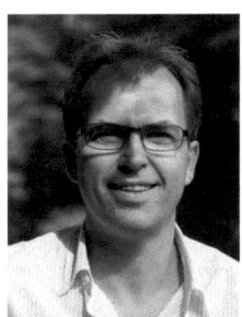 Peter Ammann is a psychologist, body worker and diploma candidate in Process Work with the Research Society for Process Oriented Psychology U. K. He has been involved in Process Work since 1993 and has worked in private practice for 23 years in Wuppertal, Germany. In addition to his practice as a psychologist he works with people in withdrawn states of consciousness and teaches process-oriented Coma Work to other professionals. For four years together with a chaplain he has been leading a training for chaplains working with comatose patients on intensive care units.